CALL OF
THE WILD

ALSO BY KIMBERLY ANN JOHNSON

The Fourth Trimester

CALL OF THE WILD

HOW WE HEAL TRAUMA, AWAKEN OUR OWN POWER, AND USE IT FOR GOOD

KIMBERLY ANN JOHNSON

HARPER WAVE
An Imprint of HarperCollins*Publishers*

FIRST EDITION

Designed by Leah Carlson-Stanisic

Library of Congress Cataloging-in-Publication Data
Names: Johnson, Kimberly Ann, author.
Title: The call of the wild: how we heal trauma, awaken our own power, and use it for good / Kimberly Ann Johnson.
Description: First edition. | New York, NY: Harper Wave, [2021] | Summary: "From trauma expert and somatic healer Kimberly Johnson comes a guide for tapping into the wisdom and resilience of the body to rewire the nervous system, heal from trauma, and live fully"—Provided by publisher.
Identifiers: LCCN 2020035160 (print) | LCCN 2020035161 (ebook) | ISBN 9780062970909 (hardcover) | ISBN 9780062970923 (epub)
Subjects: LCSH: Mind and body. | Psychic trauma. | Somesthesia. | Healing.
Classification: LCC BF161 .J634 2021 (print) | LCC BF161 (ebook) | DDC 155.9/3—dc23
LC record available at https://lccn.loc.gov/2020035160
LC ebook record available at https://lccn.loc.gov/2020035161

21 22 23 24 25 LSC 10 9 8 7 6 5 4 3 2 1

For all who dare to walk this path

CONTENTS

HOW TO READ THIS BOOK

On this journey, we will touch upon many different aspects of our humanness—our relationship to our bodies, to our psyches, to our minds, and to our sexuality. Reading this book may bring up feelings and sensations that seem disproportionate or out of context to what you are reading. This is totally normal: learning about trauma is nonlinear and can feel challenging in surprising ways. Notice these experiences, and know that they're an important part of the process we're embarking on together. Those bodily messages are helpful information. By the end of this book, you will have more skills and practice at interpreting your body's messages, trusting these signals, and knowing what next step to take to feel more relaxed, awake, and alive. With these newfound skills, you will be able to find new sources of power and energy when you feel exhausted or defeated. You will be able to discern intuition from fear. You will be able to stand in discomfort and become a force for good.

Respect your body's timing of absorbing and taking in information. Pay attention to what you're noticing in your body—your sensations, your emotions, your images, your feelings. This is the gentlest, most sustainable way to lasting, and possibly unexpected, change. If you feel restless or upset while reading, try changing your scenery; maybe you'd like to go for a walk or talk to a friend. You don't have to buckle down and grit your way through anything. In fact, please don't! Be gentle with yourself. You can always bookmark a page and return to it. This process of reading is the time to start to notice, and follow what you notice; it's one of the ways you can reestablish trust with your own body and your own somatic process because you're actually listening. You're hearing and feeling signals, and then taking an action based on those signals, which might have been something you couldn't do in the past. Now, it's important to move when you want to move. Coordinating your body's impulses with actions that respect and satisfy its needs will help you establish a new sense of safety and confidence.

You will get the most out of this experience if you take care of yourself and follow your body's cues as your read it. Put your phone out of sight, resist habitual urges to check social media, and be deliberate about choosing to read and engage in the exercises as they come. Set yourself up for success. You will also get the most out of this book if you take care of yourself and follow your bodily needs as you read it. Check in to see what might make you even more comfortable. If you're cold, grab a blanket. If you're thirsty, go get some water or tea. If you need to go to the bathroom or eat something, please do. If you'll enjoy this experience more with a highlighter or a notebook, pause to find what you need. Taking time to notice these natural impulses as you read is a part of the healing journey.

This book is meant to be read in chronological sequence. In Part I, we'll lay the foundation of a deeper understanding of our nervous systems, come home to our bodies, practice orienting inside and outside in order to feel what's ours and not ours, and learn a new language for making sense of our inner experience. Once I've guided you to establish a sense of safety in your body and a shared language for the nuances of your nervous system, in Part II, I'll help you wake yourself up out of freeze, activate your animal instincts, and embody the predator or fight response. In Part III, you'll apply everything you've learned to setting healthy limits and boundaries, creating satisfying relationships, and enjoying more freedom in sex.

As you read, you will find somatic exercises and explorations woven throughout the text. Treat them like you would a recipe. Read them all the way through first, and then go back to experience them. But don't skip them! Reading this book will provoke your mind. Trying out the exercises will engage your body and make this wisdom fully yours. Earlier exercises build on later ones. While moving through this book for the first time, it won't work well to skip around, as tempting as that might be. After you finish the book, you might find that certain experiences or sections were the most useful for you; definitely put those in your tool kit, and return to them—they will be yours.

The process I offer is a subtle, sequential approach. Healing trauma isn't a one-time project, a box you check. Do your best to stay the course, which might seem to contradict my advice to go for walks. That's what this whole process is about—navigating competing impulses and learning to understand and follow your genuine needs and desires, which shift in different situations and relationships.

Though I can't guarantee results for you, I can tell you that this path has worked for thousands of women, and it was the turnkey to my own healing that flipped everything. As I learned to listen, track, and allow the intelligence of my body to guide me, I came to realize that I had been swimming underwater and only occasionally peeking my head above. In the process of completing cycles and healing trauma, I noticed the reverse was true—that I was above water most of the time, less frequently submerged. I want to swim above water with you, and this is the way that I know to bring you here.

INTRODUCTION

In 2014, I moved with my seven-year-old daughter from Brazil, where she was born and raised, back to my hometown of San Diego. Her new school in California was a stark contrast to the one she was familiar with in our small bohemian neighborhood in the otherwise big city of Rio de Janeiro. There she would run in, hug her teachers, and fall into a puppy pile on the floor with the other kids. Now in the US, she attended a school where touching her classmates was against the rules. When she kissed a new friend on the forearm, the girl yanked her arm away in surprise and said, "Germs! That's not allowed." To soften the adjustment, we negotiated with her teacher so she could ask for or receive an occasional hug throughout the day. After a few weeks, though, her response to what she saw and felt in this new place was, "These people don't know how to love."

Apart from observing the obvious cultural differences, she was perceiving a deeper truth that has become increasingly evident since: we are a country relearning and redefining how to be together, talk to one another, feel safe, express our care, and touch one another in a way that honors our differences and respects one another's boundaries. This stage of redefinition calls into question almost everything we know about how to relate to each other, whether that's at school, at work, on the subway, at bath time, or in our bedrooms.

The #MeToo movement started a conversation about boundaries and power that has brought these issues to the forefront. Many of us are among the hundreds of thousands of women who have shared stories of violation. For some of us that means we're now reliving and living with trauma; for others it means we're reconsidering myriad interactions and wondering if they were as "normal" as we thought they were. Many others feel outraged and disgusted, yet powerless to effect change. We've named the problem, but beyond that most of us feel polarized and confused about how to move forward through gray areas where most of us are living, breathing, and negotiating relationships, sexuality, intimacy, and love. We have no shared language, no shared practices or plan for how to move forward.

The coronavirus pandemic further intensified our uncertainty of how to be together: what kind of touch and closeness was safe, how to read each other's facial and bodily cues, and how to define our boundaries. Then, during the height of the shelter-in-place orders, the murders of George Floyd and Breonna Taylor set in motion a heightened collective reckoning with systemic racism in this country. Finally, on a national scale we were coming out of denial and beginning to have long-overdue conversations about the dehumanization of Black bodies. For many, the need to participate in public protests and take part in community activism outweighed the potential dangers of gathering in a pandemic; across the country and around the world, people took to the streets to mobilize and make their voices heard.

As I write this in 2020, we are at a crossroads of redefining and reimagining how power works, what safety is, how to be together in public, and, perhaps most important, how to love. This renegotiation is happening in real time, in our every interaction from the bedroom to protests in the streets, at the level of the body. We are being called to stand for justice, link our arms together in an act of protection, resistance, and defiance of anyone or anything that would harm us. We are being called to take up space, to ask for what is ours, defend each other, hold each other, and learn to set boundaries. We are being called home to the body's untapped power.

This power is untapped because at the most basic level, we are a society that is living out of sync with the innate rhythms and needs of our nervous systems. We are steeped in a media culture that commands our attention by scaring and alarming us, a commodity culture that feeds our insecurities, and a social culture where more connection takes place online than in person. We've lost the art of healthy, civil, public discourse. We don't fully understand consent, healthy sexuality, and vigorous, nonslanderous debate. We're also deeply primed toward danger. We've normalized stress, strain, and busy, and we contend daily with other people's perceptions of us and us of them, while at the same time struggling to cultivate the space to find accurate mirrors. The cost of all this is, among other things, a profound disconnect from our innate intelligence.

I've spent the past twenty years working with people and their bodies—as a sexological bodyworker, Somatic Experiencing practitioner, yoga teacher, structural integration practitioner, and birth doula. If there's one thing I've come to understand over those two decades, it is that our bodies need us to turn inward and attune ourselves to the intelligence they offer instead of outward, where we rely on others to instruct us or alarm us. Especially now, when the stakes are so high, I believe it is vital that we return to a deeper understanding of and resonance with our bodies. Through a genuine understanding of our own physiology, we can begin to develop a genuine understanding of others.

I began my journey of reconnecting to my body with yoga. It was a lifeline for me, and over time the practice served to sharpen my awareness and provide a detailed anatomical map of the body in motion, as well as deepen my own physical articulation and experience of that map. I went on to learn and practice Structural Integration, known as Rolfing, a system of sculpting connective tissue toward greater organization and a better relationship to gravity. I spent over ten years in that body territory all the time—teaching and touching people in order to help them come home to themselves, offering experiences where people could feel how every part of them was interconnected.

Then I had a baby. Having a baby opened me to a whole new world and understanding of my physiology. During the childbirth process, I experienced an injury, and then a sequela of symptoms that snowballed after birth, as I struggled to identify what kind of support I needed and then get it. I was shocked, as many women are, at how little I knew about the process of becoming a mother. I was equally shocked at how I, with all the tools and modalities that were familiar to me, could not find the resources I needed to help myself through the process. I went through a six-and-a-half-year journey to heal without surgery, which I wrote about in my first book, *The Fourth Trimester: A Postpartum Guide to Healing Your Body, Balancing Your Emotions, and Restoring Your Vitality.*

On my way to healing, I became a birth doula and a medical advocate and translator. I studied sexological bodywork, a field of work that includes sexuality and genitals in the process of healing, as well as Somatic Experiencing trauma resolution, a body-centered therapeutic modality that helps resolve stuck patterns and integrate negative past experiences that have manifested in the body to restore the optimal functioning of the nervous system. I integrated the modalities that were most helpful to me so I could help women understand their own bodies and heal faster than I did.

Unexpectedly, *The Fourth Trimester* book signings across the country became confessionals. After readings, women lined up to tell me their stories. Often in whispers, or in tears, they leaned in to share their injuries and heartbreaks. Women shared everything from their fertility challenges, inability to experience orgasms, chronic vaginal pain, dismissive medical practitioners, traumatic abortions, birth trauma, and sexual violations. Simultaneously, the waiting list for my private practices in San Diego, LA, Vancouver, New York, and Chicago grew so long I couldn't possibly serve each person individually. It became clear to me that women around the world want and need holistic education, support, and care when it comes to their sexual, pelvic, and gynecological needs. So I decided to see if it would be possible to teach women about their sexual anatomy, gynecological health, and nervous system online. Although a strange format for embodied work, I've found there was no other way to reach more women and democratize this material faster. Now I've led thousands of women all over the world, both in person and online, through the process of accessing pleasure, awakening their power, and understanding some of the structures that are in place that make this process so challenging.

Women blame themselves for lack of agency, but these are the waters we're swimming in. The origins and foundations of the way we've looked at bodies and at healing, from religion to medicine to fitness, have been established by men. In Western medicine, the White male body has long been the standard, the one that procedures and drugs are designed for and tested on. In yoga, the male body is also standard—postures and practices are taught as if the specificities of gender would have no bearing on the relevance of certain physical and energetic outcomes. Many fitness methods, when you go back to the founders, are developed by men, and then end up being played out on women's bodies. Much of the latest dietary advice as well—whether paleo or keto or intermittent fasting—originates from male doctors and is then purported by men and studied on male bodies. Blanket recommendations are made based on their experiences, as if that experience would automatically, and by default, apply to any woman at any stage of life.

In these fields, from medicine to fitness to spirituality, the female body has been considered derivative implicitly and/or explicitly. We've begun to wake up to these biases; intellectually, many of us understand them. My work with women helps mend that divide between mind and body and offers an integrative model of pelvic, gynecological, and sexual health. Our healthcare system simply lacks the structure to effectively address these kinds of issues. Ob-gyns treat the body but too often fail to consider the role of trauma and emotions in physical symptoms. Physical therapists may alleviate pain but generally aren't trained to deal with biochemistry or trauma. Psychologists can offer useful mental and emotional coping tools, but don't address physical healing. So many of the problems that women experience are dismissed or go undiagnosed because these issues traverse many domains—biomechanical, biochemical, emotional, and fascial. The solutions lie at the intersection of all these fields: within the nervous system.

The charge of our trauma, shame, disconnect, anxiety, physical pain, or whatever issue we may be struggling with resides in our bodies. In my work, I've both seen and felt the impact of the layers of stress, misinformation, as well as perceived and very real threats stored in the bodies and nervous systems of my clients—and the very real results that come from addressing them through somatic healing practices. Most of the people who come to me have spent hours, years, or even decades in talk therapy or meditation and yoga classes in an attempt to heal past wounds, process relationships, and learn how to "be" in their bodies. So many of us believe that if we just try harder, have a better idea, say more affirmations, or journal or meditate more regularly, that we'll be happier, more grounded, and have better relationships. Yet despite the healing we may find in these practices, as individuals and as a collective, our trauma persists. Our shame persists. Our anxiety, disconnect, and anger persist. It's all the more frustrating when we know the roots of our problems, have the whole map of why we are the way we are, but still find ourselves in the same situations, triggered by the same things, reacting in the same ways.

Why are we stuck in these patterns? I believe that, in large part, it's because our default approach prioritizes the rational and the verbal. In fact, our attempts to understand and renegotiate our personal narratives in traditional psychotherapeutic models and to transcend the mind and master the body in spiritual practice have in many ways distanced us from our innate bio-intelligence, and in some cases pushed the trauma further in. Our bodies are coming around to show us that we've ignored them at our own peril, with climbing incidences of depression, anxiety disorders, even food intolerances and sensitivities, autoimmune disorders, fertility difficulties, and sleep disorders. Each of these conditions is the result of an impaired human function—digestion, self-protection, reproduction, and sleep. As a species, we are struggling with the most basic elements of being mammals.

We can't think or talk our way toward healing. Like antelopes running from jaguars, or possums playing dead, our individual and collective nervous systems are trapped in flight or freeze. If we are to move forward, we must shake ourselves out of these states. We've been taught or have chosen to ignore our bodily messages so much and for so long that most of us don't even notice them anymore. In order to feel safe no matter where we are or who we're with and to feel connected to our intuition, we need to reconnect with our bodies. We need to get in touch with our simplest and most straightforward instincts, explore and heighten our senses, and learn clear and concise nonverbal communication. We need to strengthen our felt sense of our bodies in space. What we need is to heed the call of the wild—our animal self, our inner huntress, our inner jaguar.

Of course, our traumas don't exist in a vacuum as exclusively personal problems and processes. Many of our traumas are influenced by, if not a direct result of, collective traumas. I inhabit a White body. The words "inner jaguar" and "animal" register in my system as empowering and provocative. If you are in a Black, brown, or otherwise racialized body, they may land very differently for you. Colonization depended on the dehumanization and labeling of non-White bodies as "wild," "primitive," and "animal," as a way of describing them as less than human. These words were weaponized and the consequences of that dehumanization are ubiquitous and devastating, not just in the past, but in their legacy that continues in our bodies, our policies, and our societies today. As such, the words and concepts I use are imperfect and may be jarring, for good reason. I also may make some generalizations that don't match either your personal experience or your cultural experience or both. Earth-based cultures have always had in-built traditions to integrate trauma through rhythm, ritual, dance, chanting, drumming, and many other practices. Colonization and enslavement interrupted the intergenerational transmission of these advanced cooperative practices that tended to the well-being of both individuals and groups. The fields that I draw from, as well as my own personal experience with yoga and Afro-Brazilian traditions, have codified some principles that originate from these traditions. If you are part of a culture that has suffered this fracturing or decimation, the additional layer of charge that you may feel from the use of certain terms in this book is deeply important and valid.

Learning to hear the call of the wild is meaningful work for all bodies because it is trauma repair work—in the present and for the past. It will look and feel very different depending on the body you inhabit, but the bedrock of this body of trauma resolution work is in the observation that animals in their natural habitat don't experience trauma, but humans, domesticated animals, and animals in zoos do. The process of restoring organic physiological processes is foundational work for all of us to do. The value concepts like "animal," "wild," and "jaguar" hold is in helping us imagine waking ourselves out of freeze or flight, out of inactivity or hyperproductivity, and into confident embodiment, senses fully alive, seated firmly in our own strength, joy, and pleasure.

My goal in this book is to help you heal by guiding you underneath your social self to connect with your physical self. I want you to find a deeper, inner sense of confidence and clarity that you can access all the time so that you can stand in your truth without apology, and protect yourself and your family.

I'm going to take you step-by-step through the process of coming home to your deepest, intuitive, embodied self, with exercises and a real understanding of how your nervous system works. You will learn how to listen to and use your internal radar. I'll teach you what sensate perception is and how to use it for better communication. I'll help you redirect your compass away from the fear it often points to and toward safety and pleasure.

We are at a tipping point of the redefinition and reimagining of how power works in relationships. We need new tools and a new language, so that everyone has a space at the table. We may need to create a new table.

HEED THE CALL OF THE WILD

We've all experienced situations where our boundaries have been crossed or called into question, where all of a sudden our sense of safety is compromised, where we don't feel heard or don't feel we can speak up, where the way we feel inside is completely different from what we are expressing on the outside. These moments aren't always dramatic—many of them are quotidian transgressions that, collectively, can become paralyzing. Maybe as you waited in line at the grocery store the man behind you stood uncomfortably close to you, causing you to question if it was okay to ask him to back up. Or your child kept tugging at your shirt, grabbing for your breast, even after you've pushed their hand away and said no several times. Or your partner has curled up to you in bed, looking for affection that you're not in the mood to offer, but feel guilty about withholding.

Maybe your father has a habit of teasing your young daughter, poking her and laughing every time she says stop, and when you say something about it your mother tells you to quit over-reacting. Maybe you find yourself saying yes to one more project at work even though you're already stretched so thin you're barely sleeping at night. Perhaps you find it impossible to ask for money from clients when it's owed. Or maybe the most current sexual assault scandal reminds you of your uncle, cousin, neighborhood friend, stranger, or college boyfriend who crossed your boundaries that one time—was it an assault? Maybe you're not even sure.

We've all experienced some or many moments like these: in an instant your muscles tense, your face gets hot, your stomach feels like it drops to the floor. Everything in your body says no, but outwardly you shrug it off, maintain a half smile, freeze, or say yes before you even notice you're overriding your body's cues, maintaining the facade that everything's fine. Most of us are conditioned to say yes most of the time—be nice, be kind, and be good. Be civil and keep the peace. This response is compounded by living in a culture that's geared toward ignoring the messages our bodies are sending in favor of rational thinking. The tools our society offers us to make sense of these negotiations are primarily mental and intellectual ones. Mind over matter, isn't that what we're taught?

For a moment, I want you to imagine a very different response from the one you may have felt in the scenarios above. In your mind, in your body, connect to your inner animal—the unwavering, instinctual part of yourself. Like a dog, who hears a sound far away and stands at attention with ears perked, or a cat who scrambles off a counter, able to land nimbly on all fours, you also have an inner animal. Remember yourself as a wild animal, a predator: a wolf, a lioness, or a jaguar. What does that feel like? Does the jaguar flinch or recoil inside herself when something unsavory approaches? Does she hesitate to protect herself or her cubs? No. Jaguar energy is confident and incisive. It leaps with clarity and precision, trusting its impulses. Jaguar energy is an internal sense of safety. You can trust what comes out of your mouth—your purr or your roar. You trust your intuition and you know where it is located in your body. You feel comfortable in your own skin.

This wild animal is native to you. It's in your bones, your muscles, your flesh, your cells—your whole nervous system. When you connect with your inner animal, your words, facial expressions, body language, and physical posture act in cohesive coordination. You know what's best for you—when you need to run, sleep, or play. You know that you could protect yourself physically if you needed to, that you would get out of the way of an oncoming car, or duck if someone moved to hit you. You would leave a dangerous situation as soon as you noticed it was unsafe, or store your energy until chance of an escape. When you activate your inner animal, you are able to define and articulate your boundaries with confidence—at work, in relationships, in the world. You can enter sexual connections with a new level of safety, desire, and skill. You're able to parent more efficiently with less negotiating and more nonverbal authority. You're able to stand up and say the things that need to be said without compassion fatigue or emotional burnout.

There is a way out of being frozen in fear when someone enters your physical space in line or on the train, and to feel confident and unashamed saying no when you don't want to do something. You can turn on your inner jaguar. You can heal, truly heal, past trauma. And collectively, there's a way beyond the reckoning of #MeToo, beyond raising awareness and naming the problem to building a new future, a new world together. The way out is through—through the body.

CALL OF
THE WILD

PART I

A FIELD GUIDE TO YOUR INNER WILDERNESS

CHAPTER 1

A REAL-WORLD UNDERSTANDING OF THE NERVOUS SYSTEM

A pregnant woman named Elsie starts having panic attacks. Hearing the baby's heartbeat for the first time isn't a magical experience. Routine experiences like catching a glimpse of her profile in the mirror, or visiting the doctor for an ultrasound—experiences that remind her there is a life growing inside her—are making her feel increasingly anxious. And yet, wasn't it just months before that she'd wanted so desperately to conceive?

Confused by her soaring anxiety at a time when she expected to be happy, Elsie decides to step up her self-care routine, which was already pretty robust. A longtime yoga practitioner, she takes a prenatal yoga class twice a week. She has always been careful about her nutrition—so she keeps that up, making her meals at home and adding a few new pills to her daily supplements. She returns to acupuncture, which in the past has helped her access a level of self-understanding she hadn't been able to reach in talk therapy or yoga.

Yet in spite of attending a class or appointment intended to support her health almost every day of the week, Elsie is experiencing frequent panic attacks and having trouble sleeping. The anxiety and exhaustion are so debilitating that it becomes nearly impossible for her to go to work. She hires a doula, thinking that maybe getting more of the unknowns defined and having more support might soothe her nerves. Her doula suggests that she start doing relaxation and visualization breathing protocols, and to say out loud or write down affirmations like "I know I'm safe," "I know my baby loves me," or "When my baby kicks, it lets me know he's safe" as soon as she starts to feel herself moving in the direction of panic. Her therapist suggests that she needs to sit with the difficulty—that instead of trying to solve her problems or get rid of the anxiety, she needs to be with the hard feelings. The problem is her whole day is filled with those hard feelings, which seem to be getting worse, not better. In spite of all these tools, techniques, and attempts, she is feeling increasingly out of control and filled with dread about living like this, especially with a new baby coming.

We've all had experiences where there is a profound disconnect between our instinctual body and our rational mind. We think we should feel one way, but we just don't. Our mind has ideas about how we should feel, but those expectations and theories don't seem to be getting us closer to the way we want our bodies or our emotions to feel, let alone to lasting solutions. We may have talked to our close friends and family, consulted various professionals, tried all the things that are supposed to work. In spite of all our sincere and best efforts, we're not feeling better in a significant way. We're scrambling around eliminating this food, trying that meditation practice, finding a new therapist, and instead of feeling better, we feel worse! We're more frustrated, because although we've had a little relief here or there, now we've spent all this time and money, and we're not that far ahead of where we began. Maybe this is it. Maybe we won't really ever solve our problem, maybe we are just going to have to learn to live with it and manage it as best as we can.

Every single one of us is carrying around some feeling of woundedness that is beyond our capacity to think our way through. We try to think our way out of it or meditate our way out of it or talk our way out of it. We poke at it, dissect it, strategize about it. But the truth is that we haven't been taught the deeper skills of how to listen and what to listen to, so that we can resolve it.

When Elsie called me for a consultation, she listed all the practitioners she had consulted with and all the treatments and protocols she was doing—yoga, acupuncture, nutritional supplements, talk therapy, breathing practices, and affirmations. It sounded exhausting. The schedule of appointments with no real time to integrate the support, not to mention working a full-time job, was anxiety-provoking in itself. I reflected back to how much Elsie was doing, all while pregnant, and expressed that I admired her attentiveness to her own well-being. Then I said, "You could keep doing all of these things to manage the anxiety, or you could just get rid of the anxiety."

In my life, I had also done yoga, meditation, and talk therapy, as well as chanting and mantras. All these practices helped me feel somewhat better. I loved most of them. What I didn't realize, until later, was that I had become dependent on them. I needed them to feel good. I was using them much like medication, to help me get somewhere my nervous system couldn't get to on its own. I also couldn't figure out why everyone else thought I was so calm and peaceful, while on the inside I was full of self-doubt and inner conflict. Deep down, I knew that I was a joyful person, and I was frustrated not to be able to access that joy more of the time. I had all the reasons to feel good—really good parents, a career I loved, a beautiful child, an excellent education, and everything that comes with White privilege. Oftentimes those facts that I was well aware of made me feel worse. It wasn't until I experienced somatic work—*soma* means "body" in Greek—that I knew what it was like to feel good as a baseline. The better I felt, the more I recognized the depth of the disconnection that I had gotten used to living with before.

Through Somatic Experiencing, the trauma resolution work of Dr. Peter Levine, I learned what it really meant to listen to my body, rather than to try to master it or put it into different shapes and states. That process of careful listening is called *tracking*, like a hunter looking carefully for paw prints in the mud to lead them in the direction of an animal. Through that process of tracking and locating sensations in my inner terrain, I began to feel more resonance between my mind and body. My reactions made more sense because my instinctual body and rational mind were in coordination much more often—an experience that is called *coherence*. I began to experience relief that the way I felt on the inside matched what people said they felt from me from the outside. I began to easily connect with, enjoy, and savor simple pleasures. I was able to feel when my body was reacting to the past, and not the present, and I was able to return more quickly to a baseline of goodness. I felt more like my true self.

That true self is akin to a blueprint. Each of us has a blueprint unique to who we are. As we are born and go through life, we acquire imprints. We have relationships and experiences that influence and shape the expression of our blueprint. Some experiences that imprint enhance and potentiate our blueprint, while others occlude and distort its expression so that we can't seem to consistently relate to our original nature. As a result, we live with the feeling that there are parts of our creativity, expression, and vitality that we can't get to. Or we feel that our past has eclipsed our true self in a way that feels unrecoverable. Then, we are constantly just managing the effect of these imprints, rather than being fueled by the generative energy available through living in alignment with our unique blueprint.

Imagine your true expression is like the smooth consistent grooves of a vinyl record, and the imprints are like the scratches that cause us to skip at the same places, over and over again. The imprints that we remember with our cognitive mind are examples of what is called *explicit* memory. Other imprints live in our body and our unconscious mind—those are called *implicit* memories. Most of us aren't familiar with implicit memory, and so it seems implausible and mysterious that our body might remember something that our mind doesn't. We spend our time trying to analyze and elaborate on our explicit memories, instead of accessing the wisdom that lies in the implicit memory.

The truth is that our minds are notoriously untrustworthy, our explicit memory incomplete: just recall your last couples therapy session or how differently each person you know remembers an event you all witnessed. Our bodies, however, don't rationalize, assess, or interpret, and as such, are a trustworthy record. So returning to the experience of anxiety—yours, mine, Elsie's—it is crucial to understand that the body is either responding to something upsetting that is taking place in the present moment, or responding to a cue in the present moment that has triggered an unpleasant memory or association of something from your past.

Elsie's doula suggested, after a long conversation, that perhaps a sexual violation from her past was to blame for her panic attacks. This was her narrative when we met—that pregnancy was bringing up this old trauma—and she was attempting to process this through therapy, and manage herself as a "survivor giving birth" with meditation, acupuncture, and yoga. But in our sessions, much to her surprise, sexual violation never once came up. Instead, in our first session, after I'd helped her locate a safe place in her body—she said she felt it in her back body—and encouraged her to hold that feeling, toggling back to it whenever the panic arose, she cried a little, a sign of release. I asked her if any images arose, and she recalled the death of her grand-father, which left her mother like a zombie, and her as the oldest child with the simultaneous shock, helplessness, and feeling of responsibility for mothering her four younger siblings. As she described this, I noticed her hands coming up in front of her body as if pushing something away. I asked her to track that, slowing it down and really feeling the space her hands created, following the impulse to put her hands up and push from deep down in her belly all the way out. After giving this movement all the time it needed, we ended the session by returning to the sense of safety she had found in the back of her body. Shortly afterward, Elsie's panic attacks subsided. We realized that the panic of being thrust into a mother role when she was not ready had imprinted itself deeply in her body. When that skip in the record was smoothed over as a result of her body pushing the weight of responsibility that didn't belong to her up and out, differentiating between what was hers and what wasn't, and re-claiming the energetic space in front of her, the panic dissolved.

Elsie didn't need to explore every dark corner of her psyche and try to dredge up every imprint to experience very power-ful change. On the contrary, this healing process isn't depen-dent on a narrative or explicit memory. Your body, right here and right now, contains everything you need to heal and to let go of those imprints. It may take certain conditions, and it may take being witnessed. You will have to become a master tracker of your own system. In the present moment your system is re-sponding in a way that all those experiences have informed.

Once you realize that, you can—with the practices in this book, a partner, or a somatic professional—smooth over the scratches in the record so you can finally hear your own clear song.

COMMAND CENTER OR COMPASS?

We tend to think of our minds as the command center of our bodies and our beings. Neuroscience affirms the central role of the brain with scans and mapping, while psychology suggests all feeling and behavior originates in the mind. Sensation can only be perceived through the brain first, these disciplines say. Emotion is a series of signals your brain picks up and interprets. In a culture where rationality is prized, neurocentricity rules. From this perspective, we supposedly don't experience anything at all without the brain as an interpreter.

Not only is this paradigm inaccurate; it also doesn't get us any closer to healing. It does often, however, create added layers of self-judgment, criticism, self-loathing, and confusion when we inevitably don't understand why our body is not cooperating with how we think things should be, and why we're not getting better. And "getting better" in this context usually means being more productive, "solving" problems from our childhood through analytical processing, and having more control over our minds and, therefore, over our bodies. This top-down neurocentric approach often dovetails with the teachings of positive psychology and the New Age coaching environment, where willpower is viewed as central to our ability to be happy and healthy.

What's missing entirely in this approach is the wisdom and voice of the body. While we are focused on efficiency and discipline, cognitively working through any problem that arises, the body is speaking to us in myriad ways that we often ignore or dismiss. As the pioneers in the somatic movement have so aptly spoken, the body does indeed keep the score. When we can learn how to listen to, work with, and fully inhabit our body, we can begin to heal. We can begin to act in accordance with our current reality rather than the past. The good news is that when we feel and perceive both our original blueprint and our imprints (the impact of past events), we can stop feeling that there is something wrong with us and start tuning in to the body's wisdom. We can respect our own physiology and make choices accordingly, instead of trying to cram ourselves into a model, diet, program, or method that seems to work for other people. We can witness and be witnessed in these fundamental patterns that have become the default ways we interact with the world, and then we can transform them.

Then, instead of "training your mind" or "eradicating negative thoughts," getting better might look like tolerating new environments, sleeping better at night, or forging better relationships. I realize these results may not seem glamorous. Sometimes positive shifts happen in subtle ways we don't immediately recognize. Often the absence of pain or relief from anxiety isn't highlighted as urgently in our awareness as the presence of them.

My goal is to teach you how to feel comfortable in your own skin, and feel at home in your self. To notice your body's cues and meet your mammalian needs. To be responsive to the present moment. You may be thinking, "Well that's a great idea but it's impossible most of the time. When I'm in a meeting there's no way I can get up and go to the bathroom;" or "There's no way I could interrupt someone and say, 'I need to go for a walk right now' or 'I'm overwhelmed and I need to be by myself.'" That's probably true—and it's more evidence that in every way our social conditioning tells us it isn't okay to take care of our most basic impulses. The result is that we keep getting these wires crossed—misinterpreting signals like mistaking tiredness for hunger, or thinking that we are unproductive when we actually need movement or connection, or doubling down on focus or drinking a double espresso rather than allowing for a brief distraction, social connection, or rest. Are there any basic needs you could attend to right now, even if that means putting this book down for a moment? Notice what would make your experience of reading even more enjoyable—maybe a glass of water, a few push-ups, a forward bend, a more comfortable chair, a trip to the bathroom—and follow that impulse to completion.

It may take a leap for you to imagine that a body-first, nervous system–focused approach to healing could work. I get it. It was a leap for me, too. We live in the age of biohacking, where our body has become something to master and optimize, and where everything from how we eat to how we move is aimed at living longer and "smarter." We worship at the altar of efficiency. We believe in many ways that technology is more reliable than nature, and that we can apply the laws and language of technology to the body.

The path I suggest doesn't have shortcuts, like it seems technology might offer. There is no guarantee it will take you to where you think you should go. Because the problem you have identified as being the one to fix might not be *the* problem, the one at the core of so many others, like Elsie who thought a past sexual assault was the cause of her anxiety. But it was her body that, under the right conditions, with attuned listening and curiosity, offered her a way to unwind the early associations and let go of that wiry energy that was keeping her on edge. Once she realized that "mothering" had been terrifying in the past, she could release that trauma in her body, freeing herself to the possibility of enjoying mothering in the present and future.

Just like Elsie, we're going to go through unexplored doorways to find new ways into old stuff, and this will require some trust to bypass your mind and to entertain the thought that the narrative that you've spent a lifetime forming, and may have a lot invested in, might not be the narrative that ultimately offers you freedom. You may already have an inkling that you're outgrowing this narrative, or you might just be getting sick of the same old thoughts. A body-up approach to healing allows us to move away from this fixation on thoughts and follow the body's lead. When we get closer to our blueprint, our motivation comes from the inside out, generated from genuine desire. There is a deeper underlying organic intelligence more foundational than your mind—it resides in your body, which is often begging for your attention. That intelligence is the true compass.

NATURE AS THE MASTER REGULATOR

Developing a deeper relationship with your nervous system means learning to surf the waves it generates. These waves rise and fall within us, all day long. Innumerous cycles on both micro and macro levels occur in synchrony all the time, often outside of our conscious awareness. We can learn to bring these cycles into awareness, and by noticing the little waves, we can become more adept at surfing the bigger ones when they come.

For example, every inhale is sympathetic, every exhale is parasympathetic. The potential surge of energy on an inhale is called *upregulation*, and the potential relaxation on an exhale is called *downregulation*, as illustrated in the following image. Breath cycles are an example of *ultradian* rhythms, which happen within the span of a day. Every day we also have ninety-minute cycles of about seventy-five minutes of activity, of upregulation, and fifteen minutes of rest, downregulation. Our *infradian* rhythms are cycles that last longer than a day, like a menstrual cycle that happens approximately every twenty-eight days. And we all live within some expression of seasonal cycles—the surge of spring, fruition of summer, withering of fall, and dormancy of winter. So there are infinite opportunities to live in synchronicity with the waves of upregulation and downregulation that our bodies and nature are always providing. Nature is the master regulator and lives within us as much as outside of us.

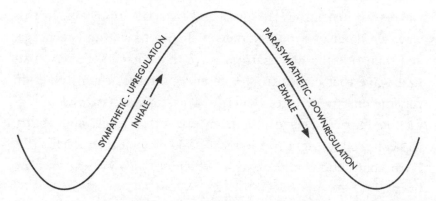

Riding the waves of upregulation and downregulation

When your nervous system is living in synchronicity with these waves, it becomes calibrated; you are awake in the day and asleep at night. You can easily digest and eliminate what you eat. Often you can even regulate your menstrual cycle. Your body is aroused when you feel aroused. You can close your eyes and rest in *savasana* at the end of a yoga class. You experience simple pleasures and have access to joy and awe. Occasionally you laugh really hard. You can easily shift your mental and physical states to your environment in the moment, and there is a grace in your movements. You have the energy you need to do what you need to do (not what you think you *should* do!). This kind of calibration is what gives us the sustained experience of—the magic of— living from a place of alignment with our true self, our blueprint.

But because we demand so much of ourselves, and we are afraid that if we stop we will collapse and not start again, we tend to override, or not even notice, when our body sends us a message to slow down. So, instead of resting for that fifteen-minute interval that we really need, we drink coffee, eat sugar, or just simply insist on staying on task. We tighten the lid of the pressure cooker. We ride up the sympathetic wave of the nervous system, but we don't ride back down the parasympathetic wave—we just lull at the peak and then ride up again. In this way, we don't give our systems a chance to rest and recharge, and then ride the next natural wave that comes—the next natural wave that comes from true energy, rather than jacked-up caffeine energy or forced energy. This constant state of upregulation impacts everything from our stress levels and ability to sleep well at night to the most basic biological functions like birth contractions and orgasm, which are also cyclical pulsing forces.

In our productivity-driven culture, most people have trained themselves out of recognizing the signals their bodies send them, considering them a nuisance rather than an elegant reminder to pause, so that they might change directions or resume. So we climb, climb, climb, and push through until we reach a state of collapse, burnout, or illness, or become accustomed to constant fatigue. Alternately, others of us don't seem to have access to the accelerator. We are in a constant state of downregulation, struggling to start our days or feel motivated, and defaulting to procrastination and sleep, as if the hand brake is always pulled.

We each have exquisite biointelligence, designed for us to live in harmony with these internal and external cycles. In order to learn how to listen to and follow our body's wisdom, it helps to have a more nuanced understanding of our nervous system—one that goes beyond what most of us learned in high school biology. We need an every-day, on-the-ground, living, breathing, felt-sense understanding of our internal wiring.

OUR NERVOUS SYSTEM RELAYS OUR SENSE OF SAFETY

I like to think of the nervous system as the main switchboard of our body. While we can't live without any of the systems in our bodies—the circulatory system, the respiratory system, the digestive system, etc.—it's our nervous system that is the command center of all the other systems. From that command center, our nervous system acts as an electrochemical operating system, communicating to us through sensations, nerve activation, neurotransmitters, and other signals how we are in relationship to our environment. It gives us information about what to move toward and about what to move away from. The nervous system transmits, gauges, and relays our sense of safety, both internally, among the other systems of our own body, and externally, to other human nervous systems. It's also a bidirectional circuit, so we can use the functions under our control—like awareness, breathing, and movement—to influence our nervous system.

A lot of what you may have learned about the nervous system back in high school biology isn't entirely accurate. Most of us were taught that the autonomic nervous system is a twofold system—the sympathetic nervous system is the "fight-or-flight" response, and the parasympathetic nervous system is the "rest-and-digest" function. There are a few major pieces missing from this understanding that were brought to the foreground through the trailblazing work of renowned research psychologist Dr. Stephen Porges. His illuminating and complex polyvagal theory, first put forth in 1994, has changed our understanding of how the nervous system functions, with real and meaningful benefits when it comes to the healing process. Once I was grounded in this new perspective, I was able to become a more accurate interpreter of my body's signals and exponentially deepen my effectiveness with clients. This layered information changed my life and can do the same for you.

Named for the many (*poly*) branches of the vagus nerve (*vagal*), the theory suggests that the vagus nerve—which runs from the brain, through the face, throat, heart, and all the way to the viscera in the abdomen—has a more central role in the nervous system than previously understood. One of the critical insights of polyvagal theory is that our old model of the sympathetic and parasympathetic functions of the autonomic nervous systems is inaccurate. Historically these two branches were not defined in an "apples to apples" manner but instead compared while in different states—one under threat and the other in safety. The sympathetic nervous system *under stress* has a fight-or-flight response. The parasympathetic nervous system *at ease* has a rest-and-digest response.

At ease, the sympathetic nervous system drives us to move and act. We need healthy sympathetic energy to wake up in the morning, to have the energy to go about our day, and to use our body in the ways that we want to. At ease, the parasympathetic system allows us to slow down, rest, digest, and sleep. You can think of the sympathetic system as the accelerator of a car. The sympathetic system takes us up the hill. You can think of the parasympathetic system as the brakes of a car. The parasympathetic system takes us down the hill.

The old model of the nervous system led us to believe that the sympathetic nervous system is generally "bad," a burdensome relic in our modern world (since we rarely have to run from wild animals these days), and the parasympathetic branch is "good." Most people think they just need to learn how to calm down or relax to feel better. "I'm in fight-or-flight" has made it into the vernacular, and is too easily misunderstood. The truth is, both of these branches of the nervous system are imperative for our optimal functioning.

There is one more branch of the parasympathetic nervous system that polyvagal theory illuminated—our social nervous system. Our social nervous system governs many elements of our relationships, giving us essential information about the world around us and, crucially, the people in it. We look to and scan the people in our surroundings to determine whether or not we are safe. That assessment of safety will look and feel very different for every individual, as it is dependent on inward factors like your imprints, as well as outward factors like your gender and race, since as we know, safety in public spaces is not just perceptually different but actually different depending on these factors.

As you'll see over the next few pages, the inclusion of these missing pieces promises nothing short of a new worldview, with at least the possibility that connection is as adaptive or more adaptive than competition—not just from a spiritual or heart-centered perspective, but from a biological and evolutionary one. Knowing your own nervous system, and its predispositions, is also a game changer. When you understand how you are wired to react, you can respond to and compose a life that's compatible with your unique system.

YOUR RATIONAL MIND IS NOT IN CHARGE OF YOUR NERVOUS SYSTEM

When our system feels safe, without the perception or the memory of threat, we feel good, and our bodies can function optimally. When our system is under threat, however, our sympathetic nervous system is wired to either move toward or away from the threat. Moving toward the threat and moving into interaction with the threat is called the "fight" response. Moving away or escaping the threat is called a "flight" response.

If for any reason a threat registers as beyond our capacity to escape, our parasympathetic nervous system will go into a low-level "freeze." Remember that the freeze response can manifest as an inability to speak, to move, or to act. We literally become the deer in the headlights. If the threat registers at a high level, one might collapse and shut down, which could look like the deer frozen in place, or fainting, dissociating, wetting your pants, or evacuating your bowels.

What's fascinating, and also incredibly important to know, is that the intensity that a threat registers in someone's nervous system is not necessarily proportional to the *actual* threat. What that means is that, from the outside, we can't accurately evaluate the size of the threat to the individual who is experiencing it. Where for one person, going to a hospital is no big deal, for another, the mere mention of a doctor makes their heart palpitate. For yet another person, the thought of walking into the hospital building drains the blood from their face. Likewise, an interpersonal conflict might be routine for one person, while someone else might dread such an exchange for weeks before the conversation even takes place. Another example is that the experience of a natural disaster or death can linger on for years in one person's system; others are able to move forward in a short amount of time. *Any* experience can register as a threat from the inside, no matter how it looks from the outside. Your nervous system's assessment of these situations is unique to you, and this has huge implications as you learn to listen to, translate, and not judge your body's reactions.

When your system is under threat, your response is not voluntary—your rational mind is not doing the choosing. You don't *decide* to fight, flee, freeze, or collapse. Your nervous system responds with the capacity it has in that moment, based on how it's been conditioned by past experiences, what was modeled to you as a child, what you've tried before that worked or didn't work, and where you have gotten stuck in a rut.

This is not a moral issue. Whatever your habitual response is to a situation doesn't mean you're weaker or stronger than someone else—it simply reflects what your system has been primed to do. If you just let that information in for a moment, yes, breathe it in, and "savor" it right now as you read this, you might feel the sweet relief of knowing that your nervous system is more consistent and reliable and intelligent than you ever knew. (And that there is nothing wrong with you!)

I once had a student who had been held up at gunpoint. The friend she was with fought back and tried to grab her purse from their attacker, while my student froze and wet her pants. The story she told herself was that she'd had an upbringing with very little adversity, and so she was "wimpy" as a result. In her mind, her friend was tough and she was weak and would fold under pressure.

Then she completed my course, learning to track and respond to her nervous system, the same way we'll do together in the chapters to come. She told me that one day shortly afterward, she was riding her bike across a bridge when a passing car almost clipped her. Instead of freezing, she found herself full of anger and ready to defend herself (she let the driver of the car know as much with her words and gestures). Her response startled her, but she realized that her instinctive reaction to danger had shifted, and she felt powerful and fierce. She had successfully repatterned her default stress response, and as a result her story about who she is changed as well. She also gained a deeper understanding of and compassion for her past freeze response.

Our systems may have become habituated, yes, and identifying our default responses is a first step. Then we begin restoring the most effective responses possible for any given situation, responses that are built in to our nervous system waiting to be ignited. We can live and thrive into a healthy nervous system. That's what this book will help you do.

MISSING PIECE: THE SOCIAL ENGAGEMENT SYSTEM

Our understanding of the social engagement system has only been in circulation since the development of polyvagal theory in 1994. Remember that polyvagal theory brought to the forefront the idea that our autonomic (the sympathetic and parasympathetic) nervous system is not an either/or, brake/accelerator system, as had previously been thought, and taught. Instead our autonomic nervous system is much more nuanced and actually works in a cascading fashion.

Our first level of detection of safety comes through the social nervous system. We look naturally to other people and go toward them to feel safe or to know if we are safe. Put in the simplest way, this means that we are always scanning people's facial expressions to determine if we are safe. This is one of the reasons why, during the COVID-19 crisis, many people have found it disconcerting to interact with masks on. More than half of people's facial expressions, that we innately rely on to decide if we are safe, were concealed.

It also means that under threat of a pandemic, our instinct would be to pull people closer to us. At a time when our body and nervous system would want proximity and support most, our mind knew that we needed to remain physically distant. Our instinctual physical impulse to come closer had to be continuously managed or thwarted. Even though our rational minds understood the logic, that unfulfilled instinct lives on in our bodies as tension and, for many, trauma.

Our most basic instinct is not "to each their own"; our biological survival imperative is togetherness and physical proximity. If there's a loud noise in a movie theater, we jump toward the person next to us. If you were camping with a group of families and you heard a distant rumble in intensity sounding like a stampede was approaching (work with me here), you would get closer to each other, pile into one of your tents, or go to the person's vehicle that was the biggest. Instinctively you would do that even if you didn't know the other people, because that would be the safest option—to be together. You may be thinking, "Nope, not me, I would go it alone." That may be true for some people (and tendencies here may be rooted in attachment styles, which we will cover in chapter 8), but if your impulse is to go it alone all the time, then you are working against your social engagement system, which is designed to provide you with a sense of safety, protection, and belonging. Repair involves respecting your real-time needs as well as reestablishing a sense of trust and safety *with* people.

Our social nervous system is the newest branch of the autonomic nervous system *phylogenetically*, which means that evolutionarily it developed most recently. In fact, the social nervous system is specific to mammals (quick biology brush-up: what makes an animal a mammal is that it is warm-blooded, births live young, and lactates). This most modern nervous system was evolution's way of hardwiring a mother's loyalty, so that it wouldn't be left to chance if she would care for her young, who are totally dependent on her for their survival (unlike other species). The development of the social engagement system enabled maternal bonding and social cooperation by way of facial expressions. A mother's facial expressions and responsiveness to her baby's needs is called accurate, or *attuned*, mirroring, and teaches a baby over time how to react to and interact with the world.

Thus the social nervous system is primed through encounters first with our primary caregiver, usually our mother or the person who fed us, and then through the rest of our family system and the other people who formed our communities, as well as all our friendships and relationships throughout our lives. This system holds our primary imprint of whether or not the world is safe, it tells us if we belong or don't belong, and it also signals a person's trustworthiness. It's why the bond through pregnancy with mother and baby and in the early nonverbal years is so critical to the development of the social nervous system. The social nervous system literally teaches us to bond, to interact, to read facial cues, to empathize, to play, to talk, and to be social beings. It also holds all our subsequent imprints of "fitting in" (or not), equally powerful imprints such as betrayal or belonging, and registers how we need to act or behave to get our needs met.

The social engagement system is our orienting apparatus and relates to our sensory organs—our eyes, mouth, ears, tongue, as well as our neck muscles that let us turn our head so that we can look around us and either confirm or deny the safety we've perceived in the environment through our senses. It's not just what we're feeling that gives us information, it's also being able to visually confirm whether or not we are safe, and to confirm where we are.

The social engagement system helps us to understand human behaviors that can be confusing at first glance. A classic example of this is when a woman returns to a relationship that is unhealthy and possibly dangerous. It might seem illogical that she is continuing to stay close to a threat, but from the "point of view" of the social engagement system, when a threat is closer, it's more predictable; it's a known factor. So if our system is not sure that we can survive a confrontation, then it's "safer" to keep the threat/person close enough to monitor. There's a kind of "intelligence" here, even if we are not truly safe. Once more, this is not a moral issue!

In trauma studies, we have tended to regard the nervous system as sex and gender neutral. However, I believe that because women, on average, have far more estrogen than most men do, women are disproportionately impacted by the social nervous system, both its strengths and weaknesses. Estrogen is a bonding hormone that primes us to be perceptive and attuned to other people's experiences. This awareness of and care for social bonds is crucial for the survival of our species and is an extraordinary gift. It evolved so that we would take exquisite care of our young.

That said, there are downsides to our bonding superpowers. We are more susceptible to the social nervous system reactions under stress—both fitting in and fawning. Women are often more prone to social comparison, concerned about how our actions are or will be perceived, and hung up on friendship and relationship problems. We can minimize our perspectives, opinions, intelligence, and aspirations to keep the peace or maintain the status quo of our relationships, family, or work life. These concerns about belonging can become deafening and keep us in unhealthy situations—whether they're dates or jobs or marriages—way longer than we might like or might be good for us, because we are afraid to break connection, to not be liked, to be labeled a tease, demanding, selfish, or bitchy. We are hardwired to care more about connection and be more socially invested in our relationships than men are. A better understanding of the impact of hormones could also help us understand some of these behaviors. In the meantime, we can also develop considerable agency when we examine our relationship to social norms, which may be operating to create some level of primal safety but may not be serving our best interests and our true, long-term safety and well-being. In chapter 7, we will dive deeply into how we can strengthen our relational superpowers while disarming the parts of the social nervous system that hold us back and keep us small.

This is critical to understand. Women are confused as to why they went along with their doctor's recommendation when it didn't feel right, or stayed with an abusive partner, or had sex again with someone who violated them. Yes, our conditioning to be "good," "nice," and not disruptive comes into play here, but so does our internal sense of survival, which tells us that we may not survive separation or conflict. Many women have gone back to their abusers, back into situations where abuse was likely to continue, or simply remained in dangerous environments even though they knew it was unhealthy. It makes no logical sense; why would we do that to ourselves? But the social nervous system sometimes compels us to pull threats closer, and we feel "safer" with proximity to a known threat than with one that is lurking somewhere out in the world.

Have you ever felt like you just couldn't have a difficult conversation, even with someone you loved and trusted? You waited and waited, because that interpersonal conflict seemed like such a big deal you could barely handle it? Beneath the fear of confrontation or conflict might also be a fear of losing that connection, and depending on your past history of belonging and attachment, it can feel incredibly scary and difficult to end a relationship. Similarly, consider a more extreme situation in which a woman finds herself afraid for her physical safety, where someone has power over her. Her desire to please and re-main socially connected can override her deeper impulses and instincts, and ultimately that can lead to a lot of shame and blame. She will ask herself questions like "Why didn't I speak up? Protect myself? Get away? Fight?" Once again, it is essential that we women remember this is not a moral issue; we need to learn about, respect, and have compassion for the survival mech-anisms of this complex social nervous system of ours. The more we understand, the more power, more choices, and more true safety is available to us.

Being attuned to our social environment is important. Can you imagine if no one paid attention to how their actions impacted others? We'd all be terrible neighbors. That's not a world we want to live in. However, many women err on the side of taking up less space, remaining quiet, becoming invisible, swallowing their needs so as not to create waves or conflict. We unconsciously choose these behaviors, which become habits, and personality styles, because conflict can threaten the intactness of our social nervous system that is critical to our survival.

I hope that understanding your nervous system in this so-cial context lifts a layer of confusion or shame for you, as it has for many of my students. I hope understanding this sys-tem gives you a ticket out of self-criticism and recrimination and allows you to have more forgiveness, understanding, and self-compassion. With a foundation of compassion, it's easier to approach the completion—the resolution and healing—of these earlier patterns.

And with this more up-to-date, real-world understanding of your nervous system, you can begin to sync up your desired responses with your present moment capabilities, which is the work we will do together in this book.

EMOTIONAL SIGNPOSTS ALONG THE WAY

In order to sync up to our desired nervous system responses, we first need to become aware of the emotional cues our nervous system offers when we become alarmed. The words we use and emotions we feel give us signposts about what our nervous system state is and the degree of alarm our body perceives, even if our mind has another story. If you have ever been mystified by your feelings—like feeling too much or not enough—or if you have ever wondered why you feel some emotions, like sadness, and not others, like anger or joy, your nervous system has clues for you. The physiological responses of your nervous system under threat—"fit in," "fawn," "fight," "flight," and "freeze"—have corresponding emotions and behaviors that can help you decode what's underneath your state.

On the sympathetic side, as you can see in the following image, the emotional "fight" response begins with irritation, moves to frustration, then to anger, and then to rage, as the threat or perceived threat escalates. So if you are feeling frustrated, that is an emotional signpost that is giving you a clue to this reality: you are having a low-level fight response, or we would say that your sympathetic nervous system is *activated* at a low level. Or if you are feeling rage, that signpost shows you that your sympathetic system is ramped up, acting (or activated) as if it is under extreme danger.

Similarly, the emotional "flight" response has its own continuum. The flight response begins with the emotional signpost of worry or concern, then moves to anxiety, then to fear, and then to panic. If you find yourself using phrases like "I'm so worried," or someone else tells you, "You seem worried," you can learn to recognize that you are having a low-level flight response.

On the parasympathetic dorsal side under threat, where the "freeze" response lives, the emotional signals begin with confusion, and move on a continuum to disorientation, then to numbness, and on to apathy, helplessness, and resignation.

As mentioned previously, when the parasympathetic ventral branch (also called the social nervous system) is under threat, our response is to fit in or fawn. The fitting-in response is analogous to camouflaging. If you show yourself less and blend in, then you have less possibility of being found or eaten. At a low level of threat, the emotional and behavioral signposts begin with loneliness, move on to isolation, and at the highest level of threat escalate to impostor syndrome.

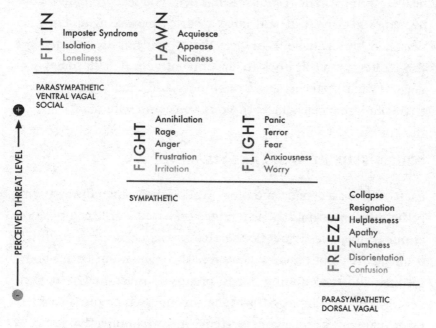

Emotional signposts of nervous system states under stress

If any of these emotions or behaviors feel really familiar to you, then you already have a clue about your default responses; and they can become as obvious as guideposts along the road of your unique journey. Some of them are key elements of who we are, how we live, and how we love. They serve us well in some situations and leave us hamstrung in others. This evolving perception of the sequences and patterns of your default responses will become a hugely important resource as a way to actually move them from unconscious (default) habits to conscious tools. Consciousness gives us agency in our bodies and nervous systems.

A *default response* is the common path your nervous system travels. If you are easily irritated, you may need help safely expressing your anger—your fight response—to earlier life experiences. If you lose things a lot, are indecisive, or procrastinate, you may need support to move out of freeze so that you can access healthy sympathetic responses that help you feel grounded, connected, and driven. If you have a hard time taking a stand for what you think, believe, or care about, you can use the support and strategies in this book to circumvent your default social nervous system patterns, and create new and vitally attuned patterns that are consistent with your voice and values.

YOUR TISSUE ALSO SPEAKS ITS MIND

Each of us has a genetic and biological predisposition toward sympathetic or parasympathetic tendencies, based on the composition of our connective tissue. Connective tissue, or fascia, is an interconnected web of tissue that weaves throughout our entire body, through and surrounding bones, organs, muscles, and skin. Connective tissue is living substance through which our nerves—what make up our nervous system—travel. Connective tissue is made of elastin and collagen fibers. We all have a unique mixture of the two in our tissue and lie somewhere on a spectrum between highly collagenous and highly elastinous; that is, some of us have connective tissue that is like a rubber bouncy ball while others of us have tissue like hot taffy. This composition, our connective tissue density, contributes to our default nervous system orientation.

People who have more collagenous connective tissue tend to be sympathetic dominant. People who have more elastinous connective tissue tend to be parasympathetic dominant. What that means is that if you have more collagenous connective tissue, you are more likely to default to a fight response. Your tissue is literally denser, your perception of your own boundaries more obvious. Maybe you like hot yoga because it warms things up so that you can finally stretch them out. You may have a tendency toward bursts of anger and your natural pace is fast. You're quick to rise in the morning, a doer, and your digestion is regular. You tend to have a hard time connecting to the abstract or spiritual—you're rooted in the material world. It's hard for you to let your guard down or relax.

If you have more elastic connective tissue, you are more likely to default to a disorientation or freeze response. Your tissue is more permeable, and so are your boundaries. You have a tendency toward low blood pressure—your venous walls actually operate more slowly because there is less density to them and the fibers have to travel more territory to contract, and create pressure to move blood. Your tissue has more space and give; you have a slower natural rhythm. You are sensitive and perceptive because of these less distinct boundaries—the literal space in your tissue for conductivity. Hot yoga is probably intolerable for you—you may end up feeling like you are going to faint or way overstretch without knowing it. Your joints are likely to be hypermobile. You are slow to get going in the morning, and your digestion may be slow. You may have very little wiggle room in what you put in your body—like coffee and alcohol. Walking down an aisle of detergents might be enough to send you into an allergy attack. It's easier for you to connect to the universal, and you have ambivalence about the material world. It's harder for you to compose and organize yourself.

Most likely you will find that some of these qualities and attributes listed above apply to you and fit a pattern and some don't. That's because we are all unique combinations of the genetic material we are born with—our native connective tissue density being a part of that—as well as all the experiences we've had and the ways that we've moved through the world. We can influence our connective tissue composition with what we eat, how we move, and the ways we engage and attend to our nervous system.

APPRECIATING THE ORGANIC INTELLIGENCE OF YOUR BODY

Throughout this book, you will be provided skillful ways to address some of this circuitry, not so that you become perfectly zen all the time—on the contrary, so that you have access to the full range of emotions, from overwhelming joy to devastating grief. That might not sound like great news if you've found a range that feels safe to you. But if you're having a hard time managing stress, or feel too exhausted to have courageous conversations, or haven't been to the doctor in years, it's likely there's some support your system could use to complete old default responses so that you can and will be available for new patterns your body and soul are aching to create.

A more nuanced understanding of your nervous system ultimately means a deeper understanding of the nervous systems around you. This knowledge won't make difficult emotions go away, but it will help you get out of frustrating ruts and repetitive loops. It will help you identify deeper level causes—and solutions—to moving out of destructive patterns that can't be overcome by willpower and drive alone. Because you have the ability to regulate your own responses, you will become a regulator of those around you, and you will be able to perceive and respond to the physiology of the reactions of others rather than personalizing them.

Most somatic practitioners agree that there's a hierarchical nature to how our nervous systems respond to threat, real or perceived. When a new threat appears, we first respond via the social nervous system. So that would be to try to befriend, communicate, or seek comfort. If that doesn't work, or if it hasn't worked in the past, or if the level of threat overwhelms this response, our next line of defense is our sympathetic nervous system—fighting or fleeing. If those responses are impossible (because we are outnumbered, or much smaller, or confined in some way) so it won't work to fight or escape, or if they haven't worked to protect us in the past (we have been trapped, cornered, or helpless) and therefore we don't have the habit of activating those responses, then we go to the oldest system phylogenetically (the one that evolved first), which is our parasympathetic nervous system (confusion, freeze, and collapse). The parasympathetic system is the most "primitive" system, meaning that even single-celled organisms have it.

If you read about these systems in most of the existing literature, this implicit hierarchy is what you will find. The order makes it seem as though our more recently evolved social nervous system is somehow *better* than the sympathetic, which is better than the parasympathetic. It seems like we are in constant pursuit of a regulated social nervous system and minimizing the impact of the other branches under stress. What I really want you to know is that whatever responses you have had to your life, including threatening situations, you have had for very good reasons. I would call them all adaptive, because they have kept you alive. We need the functioning of all these branches, under stress and at ease. We will never achieve self-regulation or co-regulation all the time. We need the clues that our emotions and physicality give us, about what is actually happening with our nervous systems moment to moment, not an idealization of how we want them to be. Your predispositions, in your connective tissue, your behavior, and your emotions are all tremendous clues on a way forward.

The truth is your past responses under stress have been highly functional and exactly what you needed. Whether or not they're functional (effective) *now* is another question. If they aren't—if you are feeling some level of dissociation between your mind and body, or if you find yourself stuck, repeating behaviors and patterns that aren't serving you—well, that may be why you were drawn to read this book. What follows is the cascade of nervous

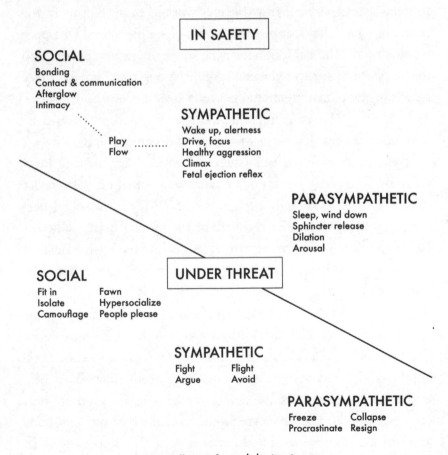

Autonomic Nervous System behaviors & states

system reactions when you are safe and at ease and when you are under threat.

At some point in your life, your system did what it could to help you survive. I hope that you can develop a continued and ongoing profound appreciation for the organic intelligence of your body, its past, and even present, choices. That radically loving acceptance of where we are now, and where we've come from, is the foundation of this work. Your job now is to start to address some of the places where your system seems out of sync with present moment situations—where the past is infringing on the present.

You now have a real-world understanding of your nervous system. As you bring the past to consciousness, through listening to the organic intelligence of your body, you will sync up with your true, unadulterated, and vibrant self. You can live unapologetically in your own skin.

CHAPTER 2

THE WISDOM OF THE ANIMAL BODY

The scratches in the records of our nervous systems, the crossed wiring that keeps us from accessing deep reserves of energy that are our birthright, are just another way of saying "trauma." Trauma is what happens when the needle skips on the record at the same place every time; the needle can't make the full revolution, so you can't hear the uninterrupted song.

Another way of thinking about it is that when we're not able to go through a full cycle it's as if the whole cake of an experience gets shoved down our throat all at once, rather than being able to eat it piece by piece, bite by bite. We can't even chew it, let alone digest the experience. Trauma narrows our vision, limits our options, shrinks our capacity, and gets us stuck fixating on ourselves rather than seeing the big picture. I like to think of the material in this chapter as a way home; it's the beginning of the process of restoration and healing what trauma has imprinted on our systems. It's a chance to lovingly self-evaluate your relationship to being in your body. We'll do this by developing our felt sense and becoming more oriented both internally and in space.

TOWARD A NEW UNDERSTANDING OF TRAUMA

I wish there was a better word for "trauma." In the age of pre-scriptions, syndromes, and prognoses, labels are dangerous. We adhere to them, they become a part of our reality, and they influence how we understand the world, and ourselves. If we relate to trauma, we may become attached to it as an identity. You might hear someone say something like "I'm totally traumatized." If we don't relate to it, we distance ourselves from it and moralize it, as if not being traumatized is a sign of strength. But trauma is a normal part of life. We all have experiences that are beyond our capacity to handle in the moment. They are "too much," "too fast," or "too soon," or all of the above.

It's important to make the distinction between capital "T" traumas—the big shocking, sometimes life-threatening incidents—and the lowercase "t" traumas. We all have unprocessed material in our bodies that affects how we act and interact with the world around us. Trauma is not a scarlet letter; it is a part of being human. Thankfully and redemptively, healing is also an inherent part of being human. Regeneration and a forward thrust of life is operating in all of us, right now.

Trauma is also not one thing. We tend to think of trauma as a specific event—like a car accident or a death or an abusive relationship—but it's not the events themselves that are traumatic. It's the way that we metabolize the events, or don't, that determines whether they linger in our system as unprocessed material causing record skips and literal or metaphorical indigestion. That's why two people can experience the exact same thing and one is deeply affected and the other is not. Two people in the same situation can emerge differently, one perceptibly altered, the other unscathed. It is also why, from the outside, we can never decide what registers for someone else as traumatic and how traumatic it is.

The subsequent residue that may show up from trauma could appear in many ways, like a twitch, avoidance of a certain place, halted speech patterns, nonstop or loud talking, eye movements or body postures, inability to access certain emotions or go to certain places, even the development of personality structures, as well as syndromes and disorders. When we are able to track and observe the places where unmetabolized experiences may be coalescing in our system, as well as make space for the underlying impulses to come to the surface, we are then in a position to allow the circuit to finally be complete. A full record spin. Wires connected. Each bite of cake digested. An ability to move forward unencumbered by the past.

BODY FIRST

To resolve trauma, we have to develop or deepen our relationship to our body. Some of you might be thinking, "You're right, I'm totally disconnected from my body." Others of you might be thinking, "Actually, I'm pretty connected to my body. I do yoga, or Pilates, or run, or go to the gym." I will caution that being a physically active person does not necessarily mean that you are connected to your body. My own experience was that even though I had spent a lot of time in the dance studio and the yoga studio when I began to do this work, it was still incredibly challenging for me. While I was used to placing and moving my body in many different ways, perfecting choreography and poses, as well as how to focus and breathe during them, I was not used to noticing how I was, while I was doing these things. There wasn't space for sensations or feelings, because what we were doing in dance was learning to override feelings and sensations in the name of choreography, shapes, and virtuosity. You have to endure pain and discomfort when you are training; in fact, part of a dancer's identity, and most athletes' identity, is to have a high pain tolerance. In yoga, we practiced nonattachment to feelings and sensations, developing equanimity toward them.

I was used to either following or giving directions and either following a teacher's pace or setting the pace for a class. I wasn't used to listening to my own internal rhythms, although I thought I was. What could have been a somatic experience rarely was for me, until I learned how to listen to and track my nervous system, and lost some inhibition about what was appropriate in a yoga class. I used to be studious and obedient, getting everything just right, focused, and maybe even a bit robotic. Much of my physical practice was still run through a mental filter. Eventually, as I began to complete more circuits outside of class, my system became more integrated, and more life came into my practice. Sometimes I would cry, sometimes I would laugh, sometimes I would tremble or spontaneously turn my head. The whole range of human expression and unwinding began to happen when I turned my attention to my body. I could allow for that rather than clamp down around it. I no longer separated my personality from my practice. I could still be me in the yoga studio, whether I was the teacher or the student.

Now that I better understand my own system, I am able to go to movement classes and remain connected to my somatic experience. Embodiment—or being anchored and aware within your body—requires learning to perceive what is already there without manipulating it. Your body tells its own story and is capable of healing.

We are human animals, and it is our animal nature that will be our salvation. Remember, wild animals don't experience trauma. Domesticated animals and humans do.

Healing begins with befriending your own body. We can't renegotiate any past experiences if there's no one home to re-negotiate them. Likewise, we can't fully enjoy the treasures of our lives without being there for them. Developing your bodily awareness and experiencing the world through it can be a radi-cal act of self-reclamation.

In spite of our body image, gender norms, or cultural and ra-cial identities, there's also a whole lot of wisdom, ease, and free-dom available to us when we start the journey to coming home into our bodies and using them as barometers for our life. It's an inverse relationship—instead of our bodies being the things that hold us back, seeing our symptoms as problems keeping us from doing what we want to do and medicating them away, we use them to understand perhaps a new path or a deeper level of resolution. And when we see and feel our bodies differently, the world we see outside of them also changes.

DEVELOP YOUR "FELT SENSE"

The term "felt sense" was first coined in the 1950s by a young researcher named Eugene Gendlin who was working with the psychologist Carl Rogers at the University of Chicago. They were studying why psychotherapy was effective for some people and not for others. The million dollar question! The key to effective therapy—to healing—they found, was a patient's ability to de-scribe bodily sensations in a nonconceptual way. These descrip-tions were often nonlinear, incomplete phrases, where the clients were grasping for words, as if trying to name something that had been previously unimagined or indescribable—something that was in present moment discovery. I would call this process a somatic conversation.

When clients I have worked with are communicating from the felt sense, they speak more slowly because they are not communicating a predigested thought. Rather, they are right here, right now, describing a moving evolving experience. They say things like "Hmmmm, I'm not sure how to describe this" or "It's hard to put words to this" and then go on to describe sensations and imagery, such as "It's like there's a grapefruit, no, it's more oval, like a big ostrich egg, sitting up in my pelvis . . ." They often surprise themselves by the content or description or feelings that emerge. As we learn to get in touch with the felt sense, the full range of experiences that are a part of the healing process rise to the surface to be integrated. Information no longer comes to us solely in the form of thoughts; we also become aware of the wider range of information available to us through images, sensations, and emotions.

Your felt sense is your animal awareness, and what locates you both within your body and within your environment. The felt sense has three distinct perceptive elements. One is to feel firmly rooted inside yourself, another is to know where you are in any given setting, and the last is to feel the spatial relationship between your body parts to one another as well as your whole body relationship to the space around you. Sensing what's originating and felt inside your body is called *interoception*, or inside awareness. Sensing what is originating outside is called *exteroception*, or outside awareness. Sensing the relationships between body parts as well as the space between your body and the room or the car you're in or the trail you're on is called *proprioception*. This trifecta of perception ultimately forms a deep sense of abiding safety within your own skin and within the spaces you occupy.

Becoming oriented inside ourselves and in relation to our environment isn't as simple as it sounds, especially in this age of technology when most of us spend so much time connected to screens going hours without looking up or looking out. While most mindfulness practices begin with developing the inner awareness and felt sense described by Gendlin above, we are going to begin with proprioceptive awareness, your sense of where you are in space. The reason for this is that if you go straight to the body and it hasn't been a safe place to be in the past, you may immediately encounter a lot of discomfort or you may begin to check out. Another reason we're starting with proprioception is that many of us already spend a lot of time literally inside our own heads, analyzing ourselves, judging ourselves, getting caught in loops of thoughts. While that is not the same thing as felt sense awareness, when we turn our attention inward we are likely to default to a pattern of thinking, spiraling toward what's wrong. Our intense focus on our individual experience is part of what can create confusion, loneliness, frustration, and unhappiness.

Our nervous system is always scanning for safety, but we don't necessarily notice that it's happening or how it's happening. Without an understanding of the mechanisms of how our bodies determine safety, we're prone to collapsing into our inner world—shutting down, numbing out, or dissolving amorphously into internal space—or on the flip side, getting stuck scanning the outer world, hypervigilantly evaluating people and our external environment.

We are able to create true safety when we are rooted in our bodies and located in the environment. When we locate ourselves in space, we can be more accurate in our assessments of everything around us and therefore more relaxed. It's a relief to see beyond ourselves—a relief to come into contact with our surroundings. We know where we are. So let's start by directing our attention to full body and proprioceptive awareness.

You can do this exercise sitting or standing. Begin by looking at the horizon with your eyes and your head. Imagine the backs of your eye sockets deepening as if they began at the back of your head and let your eyelids soften and close just a tiny bit. Relax your jaw and open your feeling sense of awareness behind you. Do you know how far it is from your head to the head rest behind you, or the wall or the bookshelf, whatever is back there? If that doesn't feel totally perceptible, then take your hands and touch the top of your head, let your hands contour the back of your head, and rub a little bit up and down. You might want to use your hands to wake up your shoulder blades, your lower back, and your sacrum. Close your eyes for a moment and let your eyes recede again. Bring your awareness into the spaces you just touched with your hands. Then notice again if you have any keener perception of the space behind and around you.

Now we're going to work with the coronal plane—the side line from your ears to your shoulders to your outer hips to your ankles. Imagine the Virgin of Guadalupe and the aura that radiates out from her. Lift and lower your arms out to the sides as if you are making a snow angel, tracing that line that divides your body in half. That plane that divides your body into front and back and that your arms are moving along is called your coronal plane. Keep softening your eyes and letting them rest back, as if they could fall back behind the coronal line. Feel everything behind your arms, especially in your torso—the back of your head, your neck, your upper shoulders, your waist. You might notice that your weight shifts back to your heels.

Allow your eyes to look around the room, beside you and behind you, above you, and below you, as you keep some attention in the back of your body at the same time. Feel free to let your head turn as your eyes move. As you look, notice where your eyes are located in your head. Where are you looking from? If your eyes pull forward, see if you can allow them to settle back. Let your attention be open and if possible led by curiosity, so you just allow your eyes to see what they see. After about a minute or so, return your gaze to the horizon. Notice how you are feeling overall, and then settle back into reading.

Millions of years ago our ancestors in the homo line walked on all fours. When they were quadrupedal, much of their viscera faced the earth. Since becoming what we would call human 1.5 million to 300,000 years ago, we've stood up and become bipedal. Our tender underbelly has been exposed and our soft viscera is open to the world. Our faces are on the front of our bodies, and we have highly developed binocular vision that is well attuned to scanning our environment—so it's no wonder that most of our focus goes out in front of us. Starting to become more aware of your entire body, including the parts that you can't see, in orientations you might not regularly inhabit, is important to developing a voluminous and reliable sense of safety.

You can return to the awareness of the back of your body throughout the day as you move through the world. There may be one cue that really resonated for you—maybe it was eye placement or heel placement, maybe an image was powerful for you. Stick with that cue, whatever it was that worked, and return to it. Notice how it feels to move through the world making that shift.

Last Halloween when I was trick-or-treating with my daughter and her friend, I had an experience that I attribute to cultivating my felt sense. As we were walking along, seemingly out of nowhere and in an instant, I looked over my shoulder, swiveled around, threw my arms in front of my body, and yelled, "HEY!" My daughter and her friend jumped back, startled by my shout, not by the menacing costumed ghost that had run up behind us that neither of them had noticed. A developed felt sense feels like having eyes in the back of your head. We are animals, and operating from a felt sense would be our normal operating zone, if we hadn't been conditioned out of it and trained to filter almost all of our experiences through neocortical activity and thought. When we are dissociated or "out of it," another way of saying not located in the here and now, our system registers that as a threat.

Your felt sense is what warns you when your hackles actually need to go up. It's what tells you to turn around and see what the noise is behind you. If you spend more time oriented to your peripheral vision and your back body, you will have less need to grip at the world with your eyes, maintaining hypervigilance as an attempt at accurate perception and self-protection. You will develop a greater sense of safety and intuitive knowing through a return to proprioceptive awareness.

GETTING ORIENTED

A main principle of working with the nervous system is what we call *pendulation*. Pendulation is happening all the time—from the rise and fall of the breath, to the back and forth of an enthusiastic connection, to the blooming and withering of a flower. As in these examples, pendulations happen at all different speeds, and at different intervals. A swing rises, suspends, falls back again, suspends, and rocks forward. There's something soothing to this metronomic motion. Every system of our body expresses this principle—sphincters and blood vessels open and close, breath rises and falls—oscillatory rhythms and pulses. Each organ has its own rhythm. While we may not be able to sense it all, we feel good when the systems are operating in harmony, like a great orchestra, all the sections playing their own parts wonderfully.

Throughout this book, we will talk about some of these systems and their unique relationships to our states of activation, arousal, and relaxation. The felt sense describes the tuning in to the orchestra that is our system. Within that felt sense there is infinite availability for perception and nuance.

We will home in on the eyes because they are so central to our everyday experience and easy to affect directly with our awareness. The main pendulation to explore with the eyes is peripheral versus focused attention. This is akin to zooming in and zooming out. Noticing when your vision is narrow and direct—laser-focused—and when your vision is soft and open as if you were looking at a horizon. Pendulating between the two will allow for system-wide regulation.

Our orienting apparatus is made up of our eyes, the other sensory organs in our head, and the muscles of our neck, which allow us to turn our head to look around. Earlier in this chapter, when you were sensing your coronal plane, you noticed how your eyes were placed in your head from front to back, and how they moved when you opened your awareness to look around at the outside environment. We're used to taking in a lot of information through our eyes. We can spend hours looking at a small phone or computer screen without lifting our eyes at horizon level or above horizon level—just think about all of the people you see on a train or bus, hardly looking up as they continue to play a game or scroll through their feed, even as they move their bodies. It can be stressful for the eyes to be almost exclusively in focused attention. Notice if that's happening right now, and take a moment to look up, away from your book or screen, and notice if your breath shifts. Notice what's around you as you open up to your peripheral vision.

There's a big difference between focused and peripheral attention, and the type of information we receive from each. When we zoom into something, our system receives the message that it had better pay attention, encouraging the nervous system to upregulate. On the other hand, diffuse, open attention tells our system we're safe. It's the difference between a direct gaze and a soft gaze. A soft gaze invites peripheral awareness. Noticing and encouraging your eye placement to center as well as feeling the back of your head opens your peripheral vision, which literally allows you to see more, and encourages your nervous system to downregulate. When you see more, you're less likely to be taken by surprise, because you can see and perceive if something is a danger. When we zoom out we can also see the bigger picture, and that literal access to a larger field often opens us up to more internal possibilities as well.

The location of your eyes may seem completely arbitrary, but actually we can use eye placement to help shift our state to more relaxation or more aliveness and presence. When our eyes are forward in the head, it also can take our head placement forward. When you are startled or shocked, your eyes widen and bulge. For some of us, our eyes are stuck in that position, as a holdover from a shocking situation, or as compensation for not perceiving the world through our other senses. If our proprioceptive awareness is compromised, we overuse our eyes as a way of gathering information. Our eyes can also be set back in their orbits, recessed toward the back of the head. That may make us feel hard to reach, and we may come across as aloof and disinterested. This corresponds to an inside focus, being less in contact with the outside world. Forward eye placement can indicate a stuckness in a sympathetic state, while recessed eye placement can indicate predominance in a parasympathetic state.

Right now, you might be furiously trying to analyze yourself, trying to figure out where your eyes are and what your nervous system dominance is. That's normal. Just remember, we are all

highly complex beings, and none of us fit succinctly into categories. That's what makes things interesting. It could be that when
you talk about certain material or a specific event that your eye
placement changes. There could be cultural elements indicative
of the place from which people in your culture relate. It doesn't
make the categories wrong or you wrong because you don't fit
them. The explorations in this book are tools to work with while
you are putting the puzzle pieces together. The exciting thing is
that we can reverse engineer the state from which we are perceiving and relating by adjusting our eye placement. In other
words, our state can determine our eye placement. Or our eye
placement can determine our state.

Let's practice.

Start by standing up. Feel your feet on the ground. Line up
the center of your feet, the center of your pelvis, the center of
your belly, the core of your heart, the back of your hard palette, and the crown of your head. It will probably take several
breaths to locate these reference points and feel a connection
between them. That connection is called your plumbline, your
vertical axis. Look at the horizon in front of you—maybe it's the
actual horizon, or it could be the place where the ceiling meets
the walls in the room you're in. Look at the horizon with your
eyes and with your head—let your chin be roughly parallel to
the floor. Let your eyes wander, slowly, without purpose or longing, at whatever is in front of you. Notice what happens in your
whole body when you open your vision. Allow your eyes to rest.
Allow your eyes to soften. Instead of going toward the place you
are looking, receive it. There's nothing to do here except let your
eyes take in the horizon of the room or the sky. Pause here for
several moments, feeling your vertical plumbline and your hori-
zontal perception at the same time.

Now, with your gaze at the horizon, let it become a little hazy, a soft focus. You might notice your weight rock back on your feet. Then let your eyes come forward toward the front of your head, as if you are really trying to see something. Your weight might rock forward on your feet. One of these directions will probably be familiar to you, easier. We are all used to operating with our eyes slightly forward or back. It does change from situation to situation, but we all have a default position. Try to stretch just a bit in the uncomfortable, nonhabitual direction and see what happens in the rest of your system. Maybe a big breath comes, maybe the carriage of your spine shifts. You can do this exercise while sitting down as well. With eyes forward, you are more likely to perch forward on your sitting bones. With eyes back, you are more likely to slouch back. Spend a moment or two perceiving the world with your eyes in the center of your head. Then let your eyes roam again. As your head moves, let your eyes stay in their new center while you look around.

Stress narrows our vision and limits what we see. When we're overwhelmed, stressed, or in freeze for any reason, we don't see new possibilities, other ways of being or moving. And the devices most of us spend our days on—cell phones, computers, televisions, smart watches—create this tunnel vision biomechanically and physiologically. Our heads crane forward and our eyes narrow to a focus on a small screen. We're actually creating the physiology of no possibility with our physical, structural narrow focus and fixed gaze. The antidote is learning to let our eyes freely roam and widen our vision. Opening our field of vision gives us a different experience of the world we are occupying. Almost all of us are looking down most of the time. In your day-to-day life, let your eyes look up to the horizon, and then up again even higher, above the horizon, every so often—an easy way to get new perspective. Experiment with this horizon or higher gaze in yoga, Pilates, barre method, running, or your functional training as well.

If you have a meditation or yoga practice, you may have trained your gaze. Your practice might have a preference for keeping eyes open or closed or some variation of the two. The assumption of many spiritual practices is that we are all too externally focused and that the answers to our dilemmas—both existential and personal—lie in our inner worlds. Therefore, in these traditions, inner experience is exalted as truth. This interoceptive preference often accompanies the narrative that the outer material world is less valuable and less real than our inner spiritual world. While I respect these philosophies and practices, I would suggest that there is such a thing as going too far inside. While most of these practices have an aim to free us from habitual behavior, they often develop strong habits in and of themselves. We can get used to directing our awareness in specific and often intense ways and lose the dance of inside/outside pendulation. As we develop our felt sense, it's important that we are able to dip in and dip out of our inner world. Our nervous system health thrives with an ability to be comfortable in solitude in our inner world, as well as in harmony in company with our outer world, and the ability to swing between them. Gaining this flexibility helps us become more adaptive, engaged, and comfortable in different environments.

In relationships with others, we sometimes find ourselves caught in another person's experience, having lost track of what's happening for us, in our own felt sense. The next time you're having a meaningful conversation, use your felt sense and orientation skills to notice how much of your attention is within you, in your inner world, and how much is with the other person, in the outer world. Give it a percentage. Can you still track your own experience at the same time you're listening to the other person? Can you notice the sensations in your own body as you pay attention to what the other person is saying and feeling? If you're seated across from each other, practice pendulating be-tween looking around the room some of the time and looking at your friend some of the time. What happens when you soften your eyes, shift your weight back, and retract some of your at-tention inside? What do you notice when you return to yourself?

I've had coaches and therapists tell me that in this practice, they realized how much tension and deliberate eye focus they were holding for entire hours, "showing" the other person how much they cared by leaning forward and hard-focusing. When they leaned back, and remembered to soften their gaze some of the time, they realized they were less drained afterward, and felt like they had offered support without abandoning themselves or overgiving. There's not some magic proportion or percentage of how much to stay inside of yourself and how much to be with another. Even 50/50 would be a big victory. It's really hard to stay inside our own experience when we are taking in so much information with our eyes, all of our senses, and our emotions in relationship to someone else—but it's possible, and it is a key to communicating honestly about our own truth, less influenced by the perceived judgment or reactions of others, which in turn allows us to feel like the protagonist of our lives.

AT HOME IN YOUR BODY

In the live session work that I do, the clients decide where they want to be inside my office. As part of our work together, I ask them to notice what place feels most comfortable, where their body wants to be. It's kind of like deciding what table you want in a restaurant. You could just decide not to care, and go any-where you are led. You could be super picky and only want a specific table. Or, if there's a choice, you could pause and assess what feels right in your body. Then you could walk toward it, get a sense of whether that part of the restaurant feels the way you thought it would, and if not, change direction and find the table that feels best. It's hard to explain *why* it feels best; sometimes you just know. That knowing is your felt sense.

We can't renegotiate past trauma or heal when there's no one home to do it and feel the way through it. Being able to recognize what is inside of us and what is outside of us is fundamental to our ability to stay healthy, digest our experiences, and have dynamic relationships. Our felt sense is the awareness of our body as the locus of experience. It seems contradictory and redundant, for how else could we perceive the world but through our bodies? However, in a culture hyperfocused on the rational and cerebral, as well as the effects of trauma and stress, living in and from the body isn't always easy or obvious.

Orienting to the environment and noticing the role your eyes play in that process is one of the simplest but most profound ways to create safety in your nervous system. How many times have you been so focused and concentrated on a task, or conversely, so distracted, that you don't even really notice where you are? Playing around with your eye placement, both focused and peripheral awareness, as well as the forward to back placement inside your head and horizon focus, can change your comfort level and confidence in public places, crowds, and everyday conversations.

Ironically, part of our intention with turning our awareness to our eyes is to notice if there is a way we could decentralize their role in our direct perception, distributing their job throughout our body—honing other ways of sensing. If we recognize when they are perhaps overcompensating, there is more space for other intelligences and perceptions to develop.

The practices in this chapter are here to help you strengthen your felt sense. They'll help you give away less of your energy unnecessarily or inadvertently, so that you have the energy to do what you want when you want to do it. Practiced regularly, they will help retrain a sense of safety into your nervous system, so that your perception of safety in the world increases. As you develop a better felt sense, you will also subtly instruct the people you interact with—their own felt sense will sharpen as they observe you. As we progress through the other explorations and processes in this book, your felt sense will provide a home base for you to come back to.

CHAPTER 3

MAKE SENSE OF YOUR BRAIN-BODY CONNECTION

A young woman named Joana came into my office concerned that ever since she'd had an IUD inserted, she'd lost all interest in sex. She was confused because the procedure went well. She felt sure of her choice and supported by her partner who went to the doctor with her. Her providers narrated what they were doing as they did it, and the procedure wasn't particularly painful during or after.

I was a little confused, too, but I also know that the body will speak and give us the clues we need if we listen. So we kept talking, and when I noticed there was a change in Joana's heart rate (which I observed from the pace of the pulse in her neck and the accelerated rhythm of her voice), I suggested we pause and pay attention to what was happening in her body. I also asked her to put her hand on her lower belly, where the IUD was located.

She said she felt tremendous pain in her right knee and could no longer feel her right foot on the floor. She was wincing; her lips started to shake and then she said she felt afraid because it felt like she had no leg from below her knee down. I asked Joana if anything had ever happened to that knee. "I had knee surgery when

I was thirteen," she said, "and my knee never really got better." She had dislocated it playing basketball. She said she never really understood if the surgery was necessary, since it didn't make anything better, and maybe even made her symptoms worse. The relationship with her doctor was contentious because the surgery didn't alleviate the pain or instability she felt. She went back several times for help, and he dismissed her, not even offering physical therapy or other rehabilitation. She wasn't able to play basketball after that, and it changed her ability to participate in other activities she loved. As Joana continued to hold her womb, she noticed that there was a coursing feeling moving downward from her knee to her shin to her foot. I asked her to stay with that feeling until it felt like her lower leg was attached to the rest of her body and she could feel her foot on the floor.

She described just how many times she tried to get help and how many ways she wasn't listened to or believed. As she now could feel a through line between her foot, knee, and pelvis, I asked Joana to feel the connection to her foot, in a rhythmic motion, pressing against the floor and softening, and pressing and letting go. "Is there anything you want to say to that doctor?" After a long pause, she said softly, "Listen to me," and started to cry a little bit. I told her to continue tracking her leg and the emotions that arose. After the tears passed, she sat a little straighter and said a little more loudly, emphatically, and believably, "Listen to me! Listen to me. LISTEN TO ME." I asked her to stay with the feeling of saying those powerful words, to notice that how she was sitting had changed, and to track what the sensations were from the inside. She said she felt a little shaky, as well as a sense of relief. She let the connection between her tall spine and her pelvis, and then all the way through her belly and her foot—this new felt sense of wholeness—sink into her system.

The earlier loss of agency and power that went along with anesthesia, surgery, and the relationship with the doctor had led to certain body parts falling outside of Joana's felt sense perception. That power was restored in the present moment as her numb or absent body parts came back to life and felt connected to the rest of her. She had come to me expecting to uncover something in or about her pelvis, and we were both surprised that we ended up at her knee—or rather, her body led us to her knee. The wisdom and implicit memory of the body gave us the path to follow.

Joana's experience of herself had been dis-integrated, incoherent—her mind and body were out of sync. She loved her partner. She wanted to have sex with him, and she'd never had challenges with sex before. Now after getting an IUD—a procedure she elected to have—her body responded differently. She couldn't make sense of it with intellectual processing alone.

Much of what is happening in our experience is outside of our conscious awareness. Connections, associations, and meanings that we are not aware of have been forged between our mind and body. Our autonomic nervous system is called autonomic for a reason—it's largely automatic and functions outside our conscious awareness most of the time. Just like my pregnant client Elsie who thought her panic attacks were tied to a long ago sexual assault, Joana was trying to interpret her body's signals through explicit memory and her rational, thinking mind—but her body was calling something else out. She needed another way to listen.

So how do we learn to listen to our bodies? It is indeed a little mysterious. But we can shake things loose by exploring the interplay among several channels through which the body speaks: thought, image, movement, emotion, and sensation, or TIMES for short.

In our human experience, we are each a constellation of sounds, signals, and shapes, in different combinations and configurations. When we explore these various channels of experience, we begin to make the unconscious conscious. We get curious about how things move through (or get stuck in) us. We develop fluency in our body's language so that we can better perceive our own experience.

Perhaps you're now thinking back to how I supported Joana through some of the TIMES channels in order to get to her body's knowing. We tracked the *movement* of her heart beating and the rhythm of her voice as well as her foot pressing the floor. We explored *sensation* in her through line from belly to knee to foot. Her awareness of this sensation brought us to the words she needed to say. Then we noticed the *emotions* that arose in response to speaking those words. This gentle, inquisitive alchemy brought forth new meaning, which released the grip of previous experiences and brought her mind and body into coherence.

We discovered through listening to Joana's body that her nervous system had *coupled* undergoing a medical procedure with loss of agency, pain, and loss of the ability to fully use and enjoy her body. *Coupling* is when channels get fused together and the association becomes so strong that you cannot perceive the individual channels. Your nervous system might couple a place with danger, or a movement or look or other sensory input with a specific experience—the smell of a particular perfume with your last bad breakup, for example. When we let the body speak, move, and untangle all the strands, we *uncouple* them and then we can see things for what they are. Then perfume is just perfume. In Joana's case, when we let the body move as it needed to, we uncoupled surgery from unexpressed pain, and lack of agency from relating to doctors and medical procedures. Then we recoupled autonomy with the body. With all of that jostled free, a new sense of safety and ease established itself in her system.

We need meaning, but we don't gain meaning from thoughts alone; we also get it from what lies beneath the thinking. Having a thought run around your head and analyzing it with more thoughts is different from having a knowing—a non-negotiable truth. Making a pros-and-cons list is different from the animal body knowing which decision is right. We may not be able to will our heart to beat or our lungs to breathe or our ovaries to release eggs, but we can powerfully influence our body's functions, as we learn to translate the languages it speaks. We have much more influence than we think. Meaning that comes to us through channels other than thought often feels more grounded and trustworthy. Something other than our thinking mind is often informing our experience, now we have a chance to listen to these other channels.

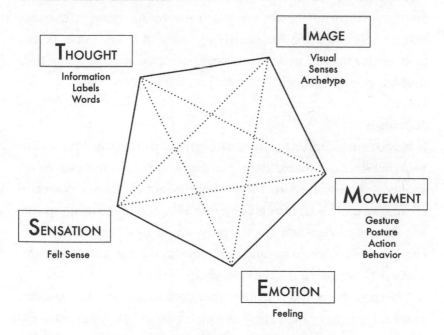

TIMES: A TOOL FOR LISTENING TO THE BODY

Thought, image, movement, emotion, and sensation, or TIMES, are the five channels through which we take in and process information. Language is linear, and so although I'm writing the channels in a specific order to organize them in an acronym, you won't necessarily experience them in that order. It's more likely that you'll weave in and out of the channels—you might find it helpful to visualize them in relation to each other, as I have in the image on the previous page. You'll also find yourself more fluent in some channels than others. Every one of these channels offers information about something that is happening within you, even if you haven't yet developed the skill to notice them. This is a process of uncovering layers that are already there waiting to be discovered, elaborated upon, felt, and expressed. As I did with Joana, you can take an approach of curiosity, start where you are, and play with changing the channels to see if that opens up anything new. But before we practice moving among the channels, let's spend some time getting proficient in each one. Be patient with yourself as you explore these channels. It takes time to learn new languages, let alone become fluent in them.

T: Thought

It may seem counterintuitive to begin with the thinking channel since this is a book about the body, but I do so because we are most accustomed to the thought channel. It is a powerful channel—our thoughts can and often do create meaning for us. Yet, we get stuck when it is the only language we speak, the only channel we are fluent in, and we confer upon it too much weight. It often belies our animal experience.

The thought channel includes your beliefs, judgments, thoughts, and analysis. Are you a mind-oriented person? Do you find yourself thinking through things or talking through things with the belief that if you just think hard enough you can solve all your problems? Is it easy for your mind to go around in circles? Do you listen to your rational mind at the expense of your emotions, sensations, or your body's need to move? If so, then thought is likely your default channel, or your "home" channel—where you live the most in your experience of yourself and the world.

We tend to believe our thoughts, and believe that they are the starting point—the generators of connection, understanding, and how we make meaning. We overidentify with our thoughts, confusing our ability to be aware of thoughts with the thoughts themselves. We love our good ideas, and feel tortured by the bad ones. We try to will away or distance ourselves from the thought spirals that leave us feeling insufficient or bad about ourselves. We make up stories about people we love that deep down we know are not true. Many of us haven't been taught how to perceive or live in the other channels, so we are limited to communication that reports information through words we believe are neutral or at least true. I know I'm not the only one who has felt sick of my thoughts, enamored by some others, but ultimately a bit helpless when knowing something in my mind isn't helping me to actually make the change that insight is giving me.

There is a feedback loop between what we feel and the thoughts we generate. Another way that's often communicated in the polyvagal world is to say "story follows state." Rather than considering thoughts to be irrelevant, the types of thoughts we have do often tell us a lot about the state of our physiology. If we are in a threatened sympathetic state in the fight branch, we are more likely to have blaming thoughts. "I don't like this teacher or writer," or "Why doesn't she just do her part instead of always shirking her responsibility?" If we are in a threatened sympathetic state in the flight branch, we might fantasize about or threaten to leave the house, job, or relationship altogether, thinking, "I don't need this," or "I'll just leave." If we are in a freeze state, our thoughts may be slow or confusing and we might think or say, "I'm stuck," "I don't know what I want," or "No one ever helps me," or we may be so overwhelmed that we can't speak at all.

Recognizing the content of our thoughts and words can help us know where we are in a cycle of activation, and instead of buying into the content of what we are saying, we can get underneath it to a subtler, nuanced layer of self-understanding. We can provide ourselves the soothing that we need, so that we move out of a reactive state. Or we can free ourselves to express those thoughts and that energy. We can bridge the gap between insight and action.

Ultimately thoughts are interpretive. We forget that there are many other ways to receive and experience the world. There are ways to experience the world directly without the intermediary of thoughts, judgments, and analyses, and often these other channels of experience give us a tremendous amount of self-compassion, understanding, and insight that is not available through the thought channel alone. There are also many ways to express ourselves more clearly than words and thoughts. We are often doing that without knowing it.

To access more of our wisdom and power, to harness and awaken our true animal energy, we must learn to move beneath and beyond the thought channel.

I: Image

Images are pictures, visuals, and impressions. Images can be externally or internally generated. If images come from outside, they arrive to us through the senses. They are what we see, hear, smell, sense, touch, and taste. We can experience them directly without thinking. We can learn to stretch out their effect in our system and savor the experience, when pleasant, before thinking and interpreting the experience. You may already know that one of these senses is a resource for you. You may feel especially connected to smells, sounds, tastes, or touch—knowing the power of one of these senses has a particular ability to change how you feel in an instant. These sense impressions become internal experiences and create sensations, generating thought streams of memories, and elicit feelings, like hearing a song you used to listen to with a past lover that leaves you feeling nostalgic or ruminating about relationships.

If images come from the inside, they emerge from our unconscious, from imagination and memory. If image is a strong channel for you, you may think of yourself as a visual person. Your world is composed of visual images—you see ideas and dreams in pictures. Your imagination may speak to you through symbols or you may see frames of a filmstrip recur in your imagination.

Images also help us to elaborate our inner worlds. When we are stuck and can't seem to get out of a repetitive thought pattern or beyond a certain sensation of pain, we can change channels to image and orient outward to an external image. We can also inquire inside and see if there is an image that precedes the thought, or if there is an image arising in our experience in the moment.

Sensory images leave impressions. Some of them can be leftover imprints from past experiences that get recalled when a similar topic or subject gets brought up. The taste of an orange might remind you of the fresh orange juice your grandmother used to make for you. And then that image that led to a thought could lead you to a feeling of a sense of being cared for or content.

Internally generated images can also leave impressions that, when anchored with other channels—the way that a certain image feels in your body, or the way that a certain image evokes a movement—can become a source of generative power for you. For example, the image of the back of your body strong like a tree trunk may serve to hold you steady whenever you maintain a boundary between you and your mother. Or, an image of the warm sunlight filtering through tall trees is one that may relax tension in your body, and produce joy, something you can return to when you feel stress. Imagery is the realm of fantasy, projection, and imagination. This can work for us or against us depending on how it is linked with our other channels.

If sensation experience (which we will get to in a moment) is daunting for you, then sensory images are your best way in. You can take an object, any object, and practice feeling it, touching it. Doing so very slowly, you can wake up your tactile sense and develop sensitivity in your fingertips. Believe it or not, this is revolutionary! Studies show that our fingertips are becoming less sensitized because we spend so much time typing and texting—in fact, surgeons are being trained differently due to a loss of fine motor coordination. So spending time slowly touching an object and reconnecting the experience from your hand to your brain will go a long way toward developing sensitivity and pleasure circuitry.

Even if you don't consider imagery an easy channel, and I don't, you may find that when you start to pause and get curious about what images may be waiting quietly for you, there's powerful information in them. Notice when you are available to your sensory experience, whether through the tactile experiment I suggested or taking some time to describe your thoughts through image. Become curious about when your mind moves into the realm of imagined experience. Dreams are another vehicle of images, so you can make a practice of writing down your dreams.

Storytelling can be an excellent way to develop the image channel, whether through listening to a story or reading one. As you hear and read vivid descriptions of scenes you have never actually seen, you can pause to notice and fill out the details in your mind's eye of the images that your mind has created to match what you are hearing. Many stories work with archetypes, tools to guide us into new insights and points of view that we may not have considered if someone were to just convey the lesson—we discover the lessons ourselves, an ancient tool of getting underneath thought.

M: Movement

Movement refers to your posture, your physical movements and habitual physical responses, your muscle tone, body carriage, and gait. The same gesture could mean two things: a raised fist might mean "I'm mad at you," or "Hell yeah, I support you," or "Power to the people." Or you might jump back and throw your hands up in fright when you come across a snake. That's also the same movement you might make if your best friend came into the room with their new baby, throwing up your arms in surprise and delight.

We make all kinds of movements each day—some are voluntary, some are involuntary. Some we make deliberately. Some we don't even notice we are making. It is the spontaneous, and often subtle, movements that as a practitioner I am most interested in. They're different from gestures, like the stereotype of an Italian person talking with their hands. Those are cultural patterns that are analogous to talking—they have a literal meaning. The subconscious movements have a specific meaning for each person, but there also seem to be some unifying patterns. Often when we express things that bring us joy, peace, and a sense of belonging we make gestures that are either opening and uplifting or midline defining—arms wide or the tips of the fingers touching. When we express difficulties, we are often downcast. However, there are infinite variations and combinations of behaviors and meanings, and this generalization isn't meant to become a tool for hyperanalysis of your every movement.

Some movements can give us clues about processes in our systems that are not complete—remnants of past responses that were stopped partway along. The turn of a head or movement of the eyes every time a certain topic comes up, or the perching forward or leaning back of the spine, the tightening of the jaw or the balling of fists when recounting a charged interaction are all examples of incomplete processes.

These unconscious and sometimes habitual movements send messages to people we communicate with and can be a part of what elicits reactions in people that seem totally strange. When we turn our attention to them, we get information about how we might, in the present moment, complete those actions. Those movements are often a little bit easier to notice, move through, and complete when we have a witness, like a practitioner, who is skilled at helping us observe the movements and feel them and perhaps their connection to other channels. Sometimes they are tiny or they are coupled with material that is so charged that we disconnect, and we don't notice them on our own. I put twitches and tics into this category of a movement pattern associated with an experience or series of experiences that were too strong to metabolize. A tic is an imprint that remains waiting to be uncoupled from the other channels involved in that experience.

Some movements are attempts at self-regulation in the moment. We usually consider these to be fidgeting—from hair twirling, playing with a ring, wiggling fingers, or rubbing our hand along our foot or thigh to thumb sucking. Those "habits" are ways our body is trying to deal with what it perceives as too much charge in the system. It's trying to help us settle by making these movements. The problem is that when they are happening without us noticing them, they don't have a calming effect. If we slow them down to a quarter of the speed or so, twirling the hair or spiraling the ring very slowly, and we become present to the movement and how we feel in the rest of our body as we notice that movement, they can begin to have their intended effect. We do begin to take deeper breaths, and we notice when the intended state is reached so that our system downregulates.

Remember the nervous system responses we discussed in chapter 1. Under stress, the sympathetic nervous system has a fight-or-flight response. A fight response elicits a front body response—gripping of the hands, tightening and shortening of the abdomen, flexion at the elbows and knees, tightening of the jaw, a readiness to engage. A flight response lights up the back of the body—calves, hamstrings, glutes, and long spinal muscles. Imagine being a sprinter on the starting block. Both of these sympathetic stress responses require muscular tone. Under stress, the parasympathetic nervous system has a freeze-or-collapse response, characterized by a lack of tonicity altogether. Because we are elegant elaborate systems, we can have parts of our body that are in one state, and others that are in another. Some of us will notice that we tend toward lots of fast, sporadic, darting movement and seem to be in motion all the time—it's hard to stop. Some of us will identify with lethargy, difficulty getting started, slowness, overall numbness, or lack of awareness of movements.

Experiences that have transpired throughout our lives can determine the way we stand and move and use our bodies. Our native connective tissue density, which will be elaborated on in chapter 7, can inform the kind of exercise and activities that we are drawn to. Similarly, the type of movements we choose, and how we do them, can help us wake up unfamiliar or dormant patterns in our bodies and be a part of balancing out our default tendencies in our nervous systems. For example, if you have elastic connective tissue, are parasympathetic dominant, and are drawn to yoga practice, you may find that lifting weights or other compressive exercises is what activates fight patterns in your body and ultimately creates a feeling of more balance and energy. There are so many types of movement—and all of them can be somatic. What becomes somatic movement is a matter of how we direct our attention, and maintaining some interoceptive awareness as we move. The nervous system benefits from variety, as it keeps our brain involved and discovering new ways to complete tasks. We can also use deliberate evocative movement and gestures to discharge stored tension or to encourage the completion of cycles.

E: Emotion

Emotions and feelings are an important part of our human experience. Feelings can be a way that we express what's in our heart, off-gas tension, share experiences, and receive the world. A full human experience includes the capacity to feel the vast range of human emotions—all of them. Sometimes we get stuck, and can only access one emotion out of the full palette of emotional colors. For instance, we feel sad a lot, but rarely notice anger. Or we feel anger and frustration, but infrequently access grief. Maybe joy is elusive.

We want our facial expressions to match our emotions. If we're happy, we smile—mouth upturned, cheeks full. If we're surprised, our eyebrows go up and eyes widen. If we're concerned, our brow furrows.

The difficulty is that most of our families or cultures didn't really permit the full range of emotions, or they had strong preferences for certain emotions over others. So we were raised learning to feel certain feelings less than others, or at least to show or express those feelings less than others. Culturally there are preferences, too. Most men haven't been given permission to cry, express confusion, or emote in a way that is associated with weakness. And as women, we're just not likable if we show scorn or anger. This isn't just perception—these patterns are well-researched. For example, female presidential candidates are coached on smiling more and scowling less because when they show and express too much seriousness or anger, their approval ratings go down.

Affect is a word that describes the combination of emotion and facial movement. Some of us have "flat affects," which is the equivalent of freeze in the facial muscles. We learned to hide what we are feeling, to show no emotion, to go through life with a poker face. You recognize that whether someone is giving you bad news or good news, they have the same look on their face— the facial equivalent of a monotonous voice. Their face looks indifferent or bored even though they are sharing really strong information. Or we have mismatched affects and facial expressions. So we say the word "no," but we are smiling as we say it, or we say yes with a quizzical look, or when we state a boundary we cock our head to the side as a friendly gesture to try to diminish the charge of the boundary and the perceived loss of connection that we think might happen by setting one, as if to say, "Don't do that, but do you still like me?"

There is another phenomenon that I have noticed over time. Most of us have a default facial expression. It's a little more intricate than the "resting bitch face." Below our expressive facial expressions, we have another less immediately apparent, more prevalent expression that people are both perceiving and relating to, no matter what we think we are projecting. For some people it's worry—a furrowed brow just below the surface of any other expression. For others it's disgust—they look like they just ate something bad-tasting. For others, curiosity or mischievous twinkling. In some cultures, phrases like "she closed her face" are used to describe when someone shuts herself off and won't let her be seen by others. While it's not necessary to hyperanalyze ourselves, it's important to know these things about our every facial expression, and it's important to understand our tendencies, since other people may respond to our default facial expression more than what we are trying to say.

In chapters 5 and 6, we will start to mobilize the facial muscles in different ways to see if we can create mobility and variety, and shake loose some of the coupling, so that we are able to either wake up the face to authentic expression, or at least relax some of the deeper habits. If your brow is deeply creased and furrowed a lot of the time, that can make you feel worried. The coupling of facial expression and feeling becomes a chicken-and-egg phenomenon. The tools of this book will help you to interrupt that cycle, and create more coherence between who you really are on the inside and how the world perceives you from the outside.

Remember the connection between the emotions and the nervous system states from chapter 1—the emotional signposts. When we are creating more balance in our nervous systems and making our way out of freeze states—for example, by saying the words we were never able to say, or completing the movements we couldn't make—we are widening the possibilities of our emotional experience. The sympathetic nervous system under threat in the fight branch is expressed in emotions such as irritation, frustration, anger, and rage. The sympathetic nervous system under threat in the flight response is expressed in emotions such as worry, anxiety, fear, and panic. The parasympathetic nervous system under threat is expressed in emotions such as confusion, apathy, indifference, hopelessness, and resignation.

In some healing and therapeutic models, such as goddess circles and some forms of talk therapy, emotions are regarded as something to elevate, manage, or even worship. Here, however, we see emotions as yet another messenger with clues for us about what our nervous system is offering. These emotional clues will help us become more resilient and have more capacity for response. This doesn't mean that we become impervious to emotional waves. Life is complex—hard things, sad things, awe-striking things, redemptive things happen. We actually want to broaden our range of experience so that we're not just falling into the pit of one of these experiences.

When we extend our range of emotions, we gain access to more life-force energy—more joy, more inspiration, more aliveness—which can become our baseline, rather than a rare peak experience.

S: Sensation

Sensations are the poetry of the body. They are a powerful doorway out of habitual thinking and feeling, and a window into our felt sense. If words are the language of the mind, sensations are the language of the body. The body is an astonishing orchestra, generator, and storehouse, and it is not an exaggeration to say that your body has everything you need to access more energy than you thought was possible. Accessing that unlimited energy resource happens through sharpening your fluency in sensation language, and learning to interpret and communicate through that body code.

Just because sensation language is inherent to the body doesn't mean learning it is easy. The language of sensation itself can be really challenging, especially if your body hasn't been a safe place to be. If you've experienced abuse, eating disorders, or a lot of physical pain, there's a good chance you've had to distance yourself from the sensations in your body. If your safe zone is your intellect, which is true for most people, have patience as you befriend your body. Try to imagine that you are approaching a wild animal. If you were trying to rescue an injured animal, you would have to approach incredibly slowly. Otherwise it would recoil or flee, and you'd have to backtrack or start the approximation process all over again. You can treat yourself with that same patience and care.

Learning the language of sensation helps us undercut the ways we normally explain how we feel, generally through analysis or feeling. Sensations are deeper and more elemental than emotions. Emotions often begin with sensation, and when we can communicate the sensation, it allows for a deeper, more present moment connection with ourselves and others with less possibility for blame and misunderstanding. It also gives us the possibility of short-circuiting our usual reactions, as we get underneath the thoughts or story we form when we feel a given emotion occurring, and communicate our sensation experience instead.

Perceiving at this level shaves away an emotional layer of shame, blame, and guilt that gets pasted over our more elemental experience, which is typically harder to identify. For example, you might be overtaken by anger and yell at your children, leading you to feel guilty and ashamed. But with practice, you might be able to notice when a heat begins to come over you, rising out of your belly up into your throat and rushing out of your head like a brushfire. As you notice the sensation move and evolve, and you even notice an image that comes with it, you may be able to interrupt the reaction, and find another channel for that sensation you recognize as anger coming to a peak. You can even describe what you are sensing and feeling in real time, which often de-escalates the situation. Instead of threatening, "I'm about to lose it," you could describe how you feel in your body. By distinguishing and then communicating from this more basic layer, we get to the core of things before they escalate, and we teach those around us by inadvertent example.

In some languages, like Japanese, describing experiences with sensation language is more common than it is in English. Since sensation is an uncommon way for us to communicate in English, I've included a sensation chart in the appendix to give you a starting point and some new words to experiment with.

You might already have a clue about your relationship to sensations. Maybe in chapter 2, when you experimented with the outside/inside/outside experience, you were mystified when it came to noticing your inner world. Maybe you just know that whenever you attempt to meditate or listen to your body, the only sensation you feel is pain or discomfort—or perhaps you feel nothing—and you've been discouraged. On the other hand, you may feel that you perceive the world very much through sensation, so much so that giving spoken language to your experience feels awkward. Either way, getting more familiar with sensation language and using it to describe your experience is critical to your healing journey, how you relate to your own body, and how you communicate to others about your experience.

When you are learning sensation language, it's helpful to start with opposites. Notice your skin for a moment. Your skin is one of the things that separates your experience on the inside of your body from the environment outside of it. Is your skin cool or warm? Is there some place that feels much different temperature-wise than another? Where does the temperature feel the best? Then notice a place that feels heavy. Pause and feel that heaviness. Now notice a place that feels light. Where in your body is there density? Where in your body is there space? Then look over the sensation words in the appendix and see if any describe what you're sensing. As you continue this process of checking in—noticing and then naming—you will open up the range both of what you're experiencing and how you can describe it.

Then start practicing saying *what* you are sensing, *where* you are sensing it, the *size* of it, and *how strong* the sensation is. "I'm noticing a spacious feeling in my chest a little smaller than a baseball at the intensity of about a 6 on a scale of 1 to 10." If you can only fill in one of these parts, great! That's a start. Remember that when the term "felt sense" was coined, the people who had the best outcomes from therapy were the ones who grasped at describing present moment sensations. To be effective and revelatory, this process doesn't require perfect accuracy. If, as you go, you notice a lot of chatter and narration, like "This is stupid" or "Are you making this up?" just gently persist in valuing an experience other than your mental interpretation of things.

Developing a new perceptive ability like this requires two main ingredients: slowing down and trusting that it is possible. The pace of the body is always slower than the mind.

Remember to Change the Channel

These channels of perception express and create an ever-evolving web of connections. We don't just explore each channel individually—we embrace the interplay among them and how they all work together to bring the body's speaking into translation for us. Our body is always communicating with us; this process is about understanding and translating what exactly is being communicated. Once we have developed this fluency with the language of the body, we can interrupt default patterns. This gives us the freedom to move when we feel stuck. If we feel mired in the sensation channel, for example, we can depersonalize the sensations we are feeling by switching to the image channel and using imagery to describe it. This often allows the sensation to loosen its grip and gives us an opportunity to get underneath it.

The process might look something like this: A client says to me, "Sex hurts." "How does it hurt?" I ask. "It's just painful," they respond. Okay, well if I didn't know what that meant, is there an image you can describe? "A closed fist or a locked door." Can you hold on to that image for a second and see what happens? Take a big breath. That door is locked. Is there is a part of you that wants to open it? What feels good about it being locked? "It feels safe and protected." Okay, so what would be the opposite of a locked door or closed fist for you? "A blossoming flower or a window with a curtain in front of it." Now I might switch again from image to sensation. When you think about that flower blossoming, what do you notice in your body? "Less pressure—my jaw relaxes and I feel like it's okay to be the way it is." From there the person might come up with a new meaning or maybe new emotions arise. Or maybe there's a movement that feels good. Maybe another memory comes up that offers information.

Perhaps you feel stuck in the same line of thinking: something like "I always have to do everything myself. No one takes care of me." Whatever it is for you, play with changing the channel next time you hear it running through your head. "There's that thought again. What sensations do I feel in my body when I have the thought? Where do I sense it? Is there an image I can use to describe the thought? What emotions are associated with this thought? Is there a movement that I feel I want to make?" Don't be attached to any kind of outcome. Give yourself permission to just explore. Let things shake loose a little. Be curious about letting a new awareness arise. You're learning a new skill to help you listen to your body and your thoughts so that you're better able to understand yourself and the people around you.

A TIMES EXPERIENCE

This experience, or meditation or exercise, is a way we can tune in and sort our own experience—a way to filter and track the different channels of thought, image, movement, emotion, and sensation.

Let's start with the sensation channel. Right now, take a moment to check in with your body. It might be easier at first to do this with your eyes closed. Then notice where your body is in contact with your chair—or couch or bed or wherever you are. You don't have to make any special posture to do this. Sometimes we're used to only checking in with our bodies in a certain yoga pose or stretch or other body movement. What we are doing now is beginning a journey of checking in no matter where and how we are, or what we are doing. Pause for a moment, feeling that contact between your body and the surface supporting it.

Notice what you're sensing in your body. Where is your attention immediately drawn?

For most of us, our attention will go first to something that's not feeling that great. A little crick in your neck. A pain in your side or lower back. Soreness from muscles that have worked hard. If your attention goes there first, that's okay; that's one layer of noticing. Now see if you can go to the next, deeper layer of noticing. Is there anything that feels good in your body right now? Openness in your chest, relaxation of your lower legs and thighs, softness in your face? If there is something that feels good, what feels good about it? What sensations do you notice? If you go back to the pain, see if you can notice it, let it be there, but shift back to what feels less bad or even pleasurable. That's why we're doing this work—to create an awareness that is larger than our pain, to zoom out, and to be able to perceive the whole picture, or at least more of it. So the question then becomes, What is less uncomfortable? What feels less bad? Where is there a positive incremental difference?

Let your mind be more like a gliding swan than a rapid hummingbird. Just notice as you're scanning around where your attention lands, and with that attention in your body, what sensations are you noticing? A tingling in your skin, perhaps. Contact between your feet and the floor. If your attention feels more like that hummingbird, then you can anchor yourself somewhere in your body: What am I noticing in my belly? What is the pace of my heart? Where does my breath move? Let the bird of your mind pause and rest or hover at a place that feels relatively good.

Now let's change the channel to image. Imagine you're sitting in a lush green field. You're leaning back on your hands staring up at the sky, watching the wind slowly blow the clouds by. And then a flock of parrots noisily but miraculously circles above.

When you picture that image, what do you notice in your body? Is it relatively easy for you to construct the image or does it feel hard for you? Do you have a relationship to the word "image"?

Then go ahead and choose an image of your own. Recall a recent memory that's not too charged, something that bothered you but not anything too annoying or terrifying—an interaction that didn't feel good, for example, or something you forgot to do, a little argument, or a missed appointment. Land on it. When you remember it, be curious about it. What image comes up? If you can, stay with that image—just one image—that captures the essence of the discord or irritation. Then notice what happens in your body. Take deeper breaths if your heart is accelerating. What is it like to hold that image and give it time and give it space?

Let's switch to movement. Notice how you're sitting or standing or however your body is positioned. Now go ahead and choose a different way of sitting or standing. First take a moment and shake your head or your hands or legs and then let your body naturally reorganize itself into a position that feels good. So rather than trying to sit up straight or have perfect posture, see if you can simply come back to being comfortable and quiet.

Now let's look at emotion. How are you feeling with respect to your emotions right now? Is there joy? Happiness? Anger? Sadness? Excitement? Resignation? Are you aware of the tone of your emotional state?

For the purpose of this tracking exercise we don't have to go too deep into the thought channel, since it is our default state, but you might notice if you're already looking around. You might notice if thoughts keep coming up. If so, spend some time pendulating back and forth—from thinking to image, from thinking to sensation, from thinking to movement, from thinking to emotions. Notice the space between, that there is differentiation between them. Then, if you loosened the grip of your brain and expanded your awareness horizontally—supposing you couldn't use words to describe that feeling or that sensation—what would the image be to describe it? If you could expand that feeling or sensation or image into movement, what movement would you make? Go ahead and slowly make it. What movement would express the image or sensation or the emotion?

Then just tuning to your original movement, take in all of yourself and notice how you feel overall. When you parse out your state of being in this way, do you feel more coherence? Can you experience yourself and the world with greater clarity? Just notice. There is no right or wrong answer.

PART II

HEALING TRAUMA STARTS IN THE BODY

CHAPTER 4

LEARN HOW TO FEEL GOOD

We are a culture addicted to intensity. If a little is good, more must be better. It's our puritanical inheritance: we're not supposed to feel good. We're supposed to be humble and stoic and work hard. But this mentality has extended far beyond our puritanical "more work is better" ethic—it's a deeply foundational part of how we approach health, relationships, and sexuality. CrossFit, paleo, unassisted birth; we are always looking to increase the stakes and maximize our time. It's not that there's anything wrong with intense experiences, but consciously or not, we've all bought into the idea that to find pleasure or to heal we need to push beyond what we thought was humanly possible. We think in order to change we need to go harder instead of learning how to settle into what feels good. Often we approach therapy in the same way—our highly activated nervous systems prompt us to go digging around the dark corners for "what's really wrong," painfully excavating every moment of our lives in a never-ending search for meaning. The result of all this focus on intensity and achievement is that many of us don't actually know how to feel good, and you have to be able to sense what feels good in order to do any healing of trauma.

What if we could learn to experience simple pleasures without needing to amp up the intensity level? What if we could heal more by pushing less? What if we could learn to *reside* in pleasure? Then when we do go toward intense experiences, it's because we want to, not because we think we have to. Rather than craving more intensity, pointing ourselves to the next mountaintop challenge or dark corner, we feel satisfied and content. Instead of the intensity sending us on a search for more, or the peak experiences leading to crashes afterward, we are able to expand our capacity to savor simple pleasures. We learn to feel satiated with less effort.

In order to reside in pleasure we must be able to perceive what is pleasurable—we have to learn how to feel good. I'm not talking about positive psychology or a reductive, naive, "look on the bright side" approach. I'm also not suggesting that residing in pleasure means hiding your head in the sand, ignoring the very real pain and oppression in the world. I'm talking about real, true rootedness in pleasure: allowing for what feels good and being able to stay there, even while acknowledging pain. This stabilization, this not pushing through to the next big thing, is in fact what expands our capacity for more. A baseline in pleasure leads to the possibility of positive reparative experiences, so that the very thing that once felt scary or even traumatizing, like a Pap smear or a difficult conversation, can actually become a tool on the path of healing.

To find this we need to cultivate perspective—literally learning how to zoom in and zoom out, noticing the things that do work for us and being able to "land" them in our systems. When I ask students in my classes to notice something in their bodies that feels good, so often the response I get is "nothing feels good." We need to create capacity in our nervous systems so that we build tolerance for goodness and joy, not just acceptance of what isn't working or a tolerance of pain. We need to stretch our upper limit of pleasure. We need to permit ourselves to do what seems indulgent. This doesn't mean prioritizing pleasure all the time; it means allowing yourself to truly savor a meal that tastes good to you, or sinking into a warm hug, or listening to your favorite song and feeling your feet tapping. The sound of the rain. Your favorite sweater. Whatever it is for you, can you put your attention there and stay with it?

Recently, the term "self-care" has become popular as a means of referencing how we might create more health or pleasure in our bodies. While there is often value in these types of rituals and therapies, self-care is no good if it's one more thing on our to-do list—or, worse, if it's self-punishing. If we're engaging in self-care as a "should," we will go through the motions of yoga, or a spin class, or the Korean spa, or even sex, with the same amount of low-grade exhaustion or dread—or maybe just dullness—that we're trying to break out of. Or we'll simply do more harm than good maxing out our heart rate and jacking up our nervous system exercising in the name of self-care.

What if we changed the lens entirely? What if we learned to listen to what we are really curious about, in the moment? Even reading this right now: Is there something that you find really interesting, that has sparked curiosity, that has lit you up? Where do you notice that in your body? Can you let that twinkly, or upturned, or expansive feeling spread out through your body like food coloring in water, and see if you can stick with it, even as other thoughts pull at your attention? Let your attention rest on the sensation that is pleasurable, and as you continue to notice, see if you can allow the strength of that sensation to intensify and become even more pleasurable. Often just that suggestion is enough. To invite the possibility of more pleasure increases the experience of pleasure. You may notice that your attention moves to another channel, like emotion or thought; that's okay, just see if you can return to the sensation channel. You may notice that your attention gets pulled to something that's not pleasurable, and that's okay, too. Try to direct your attention back to what *is* pleasurable.

As we discussed in chapter 1, we all have an original nervous system blueprint, the map with which we're born, and we all have imprints, those things that life prints on and in us. The imprints were adaptations to difficult situations we faced in the past—coping mechanisms and habits for dealing with whatever life brought us. You may have had a mother who steamrolled your needs and preferences by telling you how to dress and what was appropriate to eat, so it's hard for you to know what your needs are, let alone communicate them. You may have inherited the cultural message that foreplay is to get women warmed up for sex, so you feel responsible for climax always being an outcome of any sexual encounter, and a measure of how good you are or how successful your sex is. Or perhaps when you gave birth you were touched many times without warning or a clear understanding of the purpose, and now you're having a difficult time feeling safe in your body or even with your child. The messages of what hasn't been said are as loud as what has.

Whatever shape these defining imprints have taken in your life, the idea in this work is not to erase them. They are an important part of who you are, and they also carry the keys to healing and transcendence. We are, however, going to start learning how to free ourselves from the stickiness of such imprints, so that we have access to the full expression of ourselves. Their hold on us

can be loosened and transmuted into something that's more effi-
cient, requires less energy to maintain, and gives us a deep, abiding sense of vitality.

RESILIENCE IS THE OPPOSITE OF TRAUMA: THE RIVER OF LIFE

Another way of describing vitality is life force, the animating
impulse that we share with all living things. In Somatic Experiencing we say that your life force is like a river, with banks and
margins that can expand or diminish. The more adaptive we are,
the wider those riverbanks, the bigger the flow of the river, and
the more life force is available to us. When we're "stuck" in habits, or trauma, the riverbanks narrow, the flow of the river gets
smaller, and the rush of the current becomes weaker. The process of shoring up and widening the riverbanks is how we build
capacity—our ability to ride life's ups and downs, without being
fundamentally shaken—and develop our ability to handle stronger currents. The wider the riverbanks, the more experience is
available to us—more life, more resilience, and more genuine impulse propelling us forward with strength.

When you experience a traumatic event, one side of the river-
bank gets ruptured and a whirlpool forms along the edge of the
water. This trauma whirlpool, also referred to as a trauma vortex,
pulls us off course and into a place where everything feels highly
charged. On the other side of the river there are vortices of cure,
of healing. Most of us have spent a lot more time in the trauma
vortex, either because we end up there without knowing exactly
how, or because we probe around there thinking that the answers
always lie in wrestling with difficulty. The process of repair is
one where we learn to pendulate evenly between what feels good
and is working with what doesn't feel good and is not working.

In Somatic Experiencing we assign the trauma vortices—the things that activate our nervous system and register as a threat, or, simply put, the things that feel "bad"—the color red, and the healing vortices—the things that calm our system and feel "good"—the color blue. Our inner experience is always swinging back and forth from "blue" to "red." Remember that tracking is the process of paying attention to the breadcrumbs that your body is leaving you in the form of TIMES—thought, image, movement, emotion, and sensation—and following their trail. Tracking and stabilizing "blue" is the path to residing in pleasure from the inside out, reconnecting us with our own deeply felt sense of aliveness so that we don't have to seek it outwardly through ever-increasing intensity.

Think of blue and red like yin and yang, inextricably linked— all red inherently contains some blue, and all blue inherently contains some red. You'll notice this in your own thought patterns or in conversations. For example, if someone were to ask how you are, you might say, "I got a new job, and it was exactly what I wanted." That's blue. You might tell me a few positive things, but then you might say, "But I have no idea if I'm going to be good at it. I hope I like my new boss." You've just swung toward the red, toward what might not work or what makes you nervous. Or maybe you unexpectedly inherited some money and you're feeling grateful and excited until you start feeling anxious about what to do with that money; should you give it to your kids, pay off credit cards, buy a swimming pool for your backyard, or invest it? Suddenly that blue gift swings to being a red problem. It goes the other way, too. Imagine that you get fired from your job. You'd probably feel humiliated, betrayed, and surprised, not to mention rejected. But then after you have some time to process the initial shock, you might realize you're actually not surprised, maybe there were little signs, and maybe it's a good thing—you didn't really like that job anyway. You think about all of the other things you could do with your life and land in the blue. The next day, you might wake up with red thoughts like "I can't believe this happened. Why me? What am I going to do now?" Off you go, red and blue, back and forth.

Some of us live in the red. Everything we read feels like bad news. We can't seem to help but fixate on the worst-case scenario in any situation. From a nervous system perspective, when you are in a state of internal chaos or high system level activation, you will retrieve information to affirm that your internal state is accurate. If your nervous system is always sending you signals that you're not safe, you may find yourself gathering proof that the world is not safe or people are not trustworthy, and trying to enlist others into a more "realistic" point of view that the world is going to shit, for example. The world will reflect that state of chaos and high activation back to you, and it will seem like the objective truth. Your internal state will create a story and retrieve information to confirm that state.

But it's not just an individual preference or particular trauma history that keeps many of us living in red. Our intelligent systems are wired to protect us for our survival—meaning we are primed to notice the red. Potential dangers are going to draw our attention more strongly, so that we pay attention and can do what's necessary to stay alive. The problem is that all kinds of things that are not life-threatening, like our email inboxes, traffic, and daily news, have started to register in our systems as threats, and so we begin to live in a chronic state of activation without realizing it. This is reinforced by our culture; we are much more accustomed to describing red sensations and talking about red material and we tend to be less familiar with blue language in sensations and emotions.

You might have already picked up on how it is much easier for you to notice the pain you feel in your body than it is to notice a place that feels good. And describing the place that feels good requires us to reach for the sensation vocabulary (from chapter 3) that is new terrain for most of us. If you were to brainstorm all the emotions you could think of, you would probably describe red emotions first, like fear, sadness, anger, or disgust, and then you might go to the blue ones, like joy, awe, mirth, or peace.

Red is easy; red is default. We may not want to be there, but we're used to it. For that reason, red may feel even more comfortable to you. That's because it's habitual. Blue is a skill that we're going to work on together. In all the work I do, including how I structured this book, my goal is to keep my clients in blue at least some, if not most, of the time.

Often during my classes people will ask, "When are we going to get to sex?" or "When are we going to get to trauma?" I understand the desire to get to the "juicy" or "big" stuff first—to get to the "hard" and "intense" stuff. You may be having similar feelings as you're reading this chapter. But I realized early on that if we don't have a foundation where we can actually, first, be in our bodies together and, second, root into blue together, we can't go into the red. The red is not helpful unless you have an anchor in the blue. And that applies to everything in our lives. In our relationships, for example—until we have a safe anchor to return to in blue, it's not helpful to continue to go into the red.

We need a level of safety in our relationships before we can begin to expand our capacity—whether that means a deeper level of commitment, intimacy, or sexual connection. Blue can be many things: humor, play, adventure, or pleasure. In communication, blue might mean expressing the things that you appreciate about your partner, your relationship, or the way you connect, before you express what's not working and what you

don't like. The good news is that the more we point our awareness toward the blue, the more accessible it becomes. So although
it may seem like a chicken-and-egg phenomenon, it doesn't matter where you begin. All that matters is that we work together
to lean away from our negativity biases, and lean in to what *is*
working.

EXPANDING CAPACITY:
PENDULATING BETWEEN BLUE AND RED

When your nervous system is healthy you can go back and forth,
pendulating between blue and red, widening the river. If we're
stuck in red, there's nowhere to pendulate.

Sometimes we get stuck in red as a result of an experience
that feels too big to handle—it overwhelms our system. This
can happen not only with negative or traumatic experiences, but
also with seemingly positive events—like receiving the biggest
paycheck of your life, loving someone more than you ever have,
or giving birth to a baby. If our riverbanks are narrow, when the
upsurge of the river starts to get big and tries to push through
the narrow riverbanks, our nervous system only feels the force
of the surge, and cannot differentiate if that surge is red or blue.
The river then breaks through the banks and siphons off into
one of the vortices, diminishing the force and power of the river.
Therefore, even something that we think should feel good, like
a new love interest or great opportunity, can register in our system as negative or dangerous because we don't have the capacity
to handle it. If our nervous system is more familiar with being
in the red, then that's often where we end up when something
feels big.

For many people, that's the experience of orgasm. Orgasm is
pushing our limits of experience and introducing added charge

in our nervous system, or more thrust of water through the riverbanks, creating more pressure on the riverbanks. If we simply don't have riverbanks strong enough for that amount of energy, or if the state created is physiologically reminiscent of an earlier red experience, this causes us to go into our stress responses. I have a client who noticed that almost every time she orgasms, she picks a fight with her boyfriend within twelve hours. Many others cry after orgasm. There's a dysregulation happening—the autonomic nervous system is showing that there is leftover unprocessed charge from the experience that is coming out in the emotion channel as anger, irritation, sadness, grief, or just a surging of emotion. She's stretching beyond her capacity. Even though the orgasm seems blue at the time, her system either doesn't have the capacity to hold the added charge or is revealing some other information to her, and then has a twelve-hour pendulation to red. Pendulations have their own rhythms and timing. Of course, the freeing up of emotion is not always a sign of dysregulation; in fact the free flow and release of deep feeling can also be blue in and of itself. Oftentimes, sexual energy and orgasm are powerful liberators of information from the different channels, giving us clues and new windows into ourselves, which we will explore more in chapter 9.

If we can expand our capacity, or the banks of our river, and begin to move more easily between red and blue, eventually the pendulations get wider and wider so that we can be with the full range of our emotions and experience, all the while feeling a baseline of safety. Instead of the full range of emotions feeling overwhelming, it feels like wholeness, and we know how to move with it.

When we stretch our capacity for pendulation, the waves may increase, but we don't get rocked as hard. We learn to surf them as we heal and repair where our life-force energy had been leaking—and then we can listen to the news or the traffic report without taking that negative charge with us into the office or school carpool. You can keep moving forward, living the truth of your own life in the face of injustices.

ANCHORING IN BLUE

How do we orient to blue and grow our capacity to stay there?

Orienting to blue in the environment is seeing something safe or pleasurable that your eyes capture on the outside; anchoring or landing blue is being able to feel that sense of safety or pleasure through your system on the inside.

As we learn to orient to blue, and we land it, often we will experience a mini downregulation. You might yawn, your facial coloring might change, you may take a bigger breath. You may lean back a little bit. Those are all sensations to notice, so that you become attuned to these cues. Maybe nothing happens, and that's okay, too.

Allow your eyes to go where they want to. Then notice if anything catches their attention. Is there anything that you like looking at, that registers as blue, as pleasant to you? Like a bird landing on a branch, allow your attention to rest there for a beat or two. Notice what happens in your body. What tells you that it's blue from the inside? Maybe your eyes landed on a collage that your child made (blue), and on the inside you felt a warm softness in your chest (blue sensations). Or maybe you landed on a collage your child made (blue), and immediately felt heat rise in your throat and pressure in your head (red sensations) as you remember the chaotic morning you had with your child (red image). We can't control the cascade of sensations and associations that run through our minds, but we can become experts at protracting time and stalking the blue.

Remember that blue is relative. So if finding a sensation that feels good feels impossible, find something that feels less bad. You will have to practice. Most of us aren't used to registering and reporting positive sensations. The more you train yourself to notice the blue, or the less red, the more often you will notice that your attention is drawn there on its own. You'll find yourself looking up from your computer screen to take in the skyline outside your window, or really savoring something sweet. You'll notice your feet firmly grounded on the floor or pleasure at the memory of something funny your friend said. You create reference points in blue, stretching the pendulation there. The more you pendulate into the blue, the less you go into the red, and if you do go into the red, you don't stay there as long, before you swing back to the blue. Remember, you aren't trying to deny or dismiss any part of your experience; you are becoming open to seeing, feeling, and being with things that feel good.

For many of us, the word "pleasure" is not an automatic blue, and for good reason. Pleasure is presented as the antithesis to productivity, and therefore value. Many women don't feel like they are allowed to feel pleasure or show that they are experiencing it. Something about pleasure feels vulnerable and unsafe, not to mention frivolous. Pleasure has to do with being-ness, not doing-ness. Pleasure is an extra or a reward that's out there for us to earn. And for some of us, pleasure is associated with sex, or risky behavior, or financial risk, or fear of taking something too far. One of the narratives we've all grown up with is that once we get a little bit of pleasure, we'll want more and we'll become addicted to the pursuit of pleasure—we'll stop being productive or respectable and become lazy hedonists. Maybe there's even been a time in your life when this was true, when you drank, smoke, ate, or sexed to excess. Or maybe you went in the other direction, you controlled your pleasure, making sure to be equanimous and measured so nothing would get out of hand.

In chapter 9, we'll talk more about pleasure and sex, and all the things that can get tangled up there. Right now, we're talking about simple sensory pleasures. Take a moment to reflect on what brings you pleasure. Then use your image channel to conjure up that visual, smell, taste, sound, or touch. Here are a few activities that I find pleasurable. Maybe these images bring you pleasure, too, or maybe not—you can add your own images to the list below. Go underneath your thoughts and notice your bodily response—movement, emotion, or sensation—to each image. Allow for a few breaths between each image, so that you can explore how each experience registers in your system.

- Immersing my feet in the ocean or a creek on a hot day
- Getting into hot springs while it's snowing out
- Blowing bubbles into a soft breeze
- Holding hands with my daughter, swinging our arms in sync, and singing a tune together
- Biting into a perfectly textured ripe plum, sour on the outside and sweet on the inside
- Smelling jasmine on a night walk

Choose an image, yours or mine, that is your favorite. Then really savor that image for more than a few breaths. Start with at least sixty seconds. You don't actually have to have experienced the image in real life; it just needs to appeal to you in this moment. Observe the sensations and emotions as they arise in your body. When you notice your mind wandering to thoughts or associations, return to the image again. Does it bring a smile to your face? Do you salivate? Are your feet active and moving? What happens for you as you take in the pleasure of the image? You might notice that you pendulate to red. If you do, bring yourself back to the original image. Corral your mind to stay with the evolving and deepening sensations of blue.

It sounds easy, but it's not. It takes priming to both focus your attention and allow it to stick with something pleasurable. So set your timer, and decide to stick with the process of savoring the goodness for one minute. I have students who say that it is literally impossible to find anything that feels good. Every image turns red and then they can't get back to blue. Maybe you can relate to the red bias, where everything seems like evidence of an unfair, lonely, and messed-up world. This is a trauma response, and it is something that we can change. We change it bit by bit through restoring our bodies' sense of safety and trust in simple pleasures.

What we did in this image exercise was shift between the image channel and the sensation channel. I offered imagery that for most people registers as blue, or you used one of your own, and then you tracked your sensations. This is a great exercise to practice so that in your daily experience, you can also become more attuned to blue. Blue is always present, because it is the yin to red's yang. They don't exist without each other. There is no such thing as a totally blue world or a totally red world, and we are not aiming for that.

Remember that without blue, we're just stuck in red, with nowhere to pendulate. If you are a parent and you typically have chaotic mornings where you're trying to get everyone dressed and fed and out of the house (including yourself!), can you try to look for the blue in your morning routine? This doesn't mean you have to wake up early, light incense, drink lemon water, and write in a journal. In the morning routine that already exists at your house, is there anything that's blue? The way the early morning sun filters in through the window? The smell of coffee brewing? A second of quiet before everyone else wakes up? The sensation of a cold (or warm) splash of water on your face? An early morning cuddle in bed with your child or partner? I find that when I remember to notice the blue, I slow down. Then I'm able to savor more of the morning moments, chatting with my daughter as I make her breakfast while eating mine.

The next question you can ask is: "Is there anything I could do to make it more blue?" Another way of asking that question is: "How can I make this moment, experience, conversation even more enjoyable?" I call this turning up the volume of blue. Of course, there are external things that we can do, like making a special breakfast, or playing music, or taking our time in the shower. Those are all things to "do," and they're great. I'm all for making each moment as enjoyable as possible. And often it's these simple tweaks that help to amplify blue. I know I sometimes forget how much playing music shifts the energy of the room when we start our day. Why not make each moment as enjoyable as possible?

Turning up the volume of blue is in part about making these kinds of changes in our environment, but it's also about attuning to blue internally, which is an even more foundational task. Is there anything you can do from the inside to turn up the dial of the enjoyment factor in your experience? Sometimes as I'm driving my daughter to school I'll ask myself, "Could this be more blue?" A lot of the time creating more space for blue is just a matter of letting go of extra stress that I'm carrying, because I've become used to it. Our system aims itself toward homeostasis, so if we're used to struggling, working hard, and furrowing our brows most of the day, we'll find ourselves doing that even when we don't need to be stressed out. When you ask yourself, "How can this be more blue?" you give yourself the opportunity to let go of habitual muscle tension, emotional holding, or mental grinding. It's a process, and it takes time. Just remembering to ask the question often shifts our attention.

This process of expanding the blue side of the pendulation requires one ingredient that can be surprisingly difficult to cultivate: we need to develop preferences. We have to start not only noticing pleasurable sensations, but also *liking* them, and even allowing them to expand.

DO WE NEED TO EXPERIENCE PAIN TO EXPAND OUR CAPACITY?

Yes, red can help us grow. Healer, author, and trauma specialist Resmaa Menakem calls it "clean pain," the pain that's necessary to feel, versus "dirty pain," the pain that keeps us stuck. It's also called eustress, the difficult things as simple as yoga poses, ice baths, tough workouts, or messy conversations, or as complex as anti-racism work that may be hard for us but ultimately will stretch our capacity, widen our riverbanks, and create bodies and cultures we want to live in. Yet the process of orienting and landing blue remains crucial, because it's so much easier to be in the red. The foundational safety that blue offers us helps make meaningful clean pain, more possible. With a strong reference point in blue, we build our discernment so that we know how to decide the right kind of pain to stick with and track, as well as the kind of pain that we want to move away from and opt out of.

Many of us already believe that being uncomfortable brings us closer to the change we think we need to make, to solving the problem we think we have. We often think the answers lie in analyzing all of our problems and coming up with a story for

why we feel the way we do. We see iterations of this idea every-
where: "Do one thing that sucks every day" or "Push your edges,
that's where the growth is." As a yoga teacher, I saw many students (and teachers) who believed that there was some better
way for a body to be than how it actually was in that moment,
and who wanted to try their hardest to get that change. Let's just
say it wasn't really an attitude of love and celebration—and if
your yoga experience has been different, hallelujah. Almost every student could make poses more difficult for themselves, but
they couldn't make poses less challenging. Even if they knew
how to make a pose a more enjoyable experience, they wouldn't,
because that goes against our fundamental idea that if we try
harder, we'll get more out of the class or workout. Most new
students resisted using props, seeing them as evidence of being
less capable, instead adopting an attitude of "I can do this," no
matter how much more struggle holding the misaligned triangle
pose was. It seems like most of us would rather look good than
feel good. We aren't convinced that feeling good could actually
be good for us. We aren't convinced that feeling good and experiencing comfort are an important part of wholeness and could
also hold information and insight for us.

Looking for the blue is recognizing the opportunity for the
experience of blue between the edges, and that pushing edges
may actually heighten nervous system activation—the kind that
we're trying to coax our way out of. We're not used to the idea
that more ease and more pleasure might actually get us to where
we want to go, rather than being the reward at the end destination on the road of challenge. Right now, I invite you to feel into
your own comfort. To make yourself even more comfortable,
physically, right now, would that mean lying down or propping
yourself up? Do you need to let your eyes wander for a moment?
What could you do right now to feel more comfortable? Make

those small shifts, and then pause for a few breaths and see what happens. Small moments when we remember to check in with ourselves and extend loving-care make a big difference. As you continue through this book, you may notice them happening more spontaneously, as if your body is reminding you, without having to use pain to get your attention.

You may be thinking that you know people who have just the opposite orientation. They avoid difficulty, and try to get around the hard work of facing the very real challenges that life has presented and imprinted on them. To be honest, I have come across very few people like this in my work. What I have seen more of is such a strong identification with the more obvious "dirty pain"—whether a physical symptom, certain event, difficult relationship, or even therapeutic process—that it has eclipsed the "clean pain." A person is so buried by imprints and their stickiness that it's harder to get to the place where alchemy can really happen. By the time we get underneath the loudest, or most repetitive, patterns or symptoms to the thing that has been buried or invisible, potentially causing those symptoms, the process is much less painful than the person had originally anticipated it might be.

Sure, sometimes we may be unwilling to be uncomfortable. We may be operating in a very narrow zone of experience, using distractions as ways to self-regulate rather than face what feels like extreme difficulty and fear of what we will find. However, whether you plow toward difficulty or sometimes avoid it, building our capacity for blue is a necessary skill. Freeing ourselves of the grip of red requires a foundation in the blue. If you find yourself fighting this idea, if you feel like you want to skim and skip over this whole pleasure thing so you can get to what really matters, remember that feeling pleasure is a prerequisite for being able to do deeper reparative work.

Every single one of us can benefit from slowing down and letting it sink in that we are alive, and that there is beauty and goodness around us, even if we don't yet feel it within us.

IS THERE A DOWNSIDE TO BLUE?

If you have a tendency toward a glass-is-half-full coping strategy, then getting beneath that blue shellac can be challenging. Some of us have survived really challenging circumstances by seeing the bright side of everything. Maybe you grew up with parents who were ill-equipped or not around. Instead of falling into the stereotype of blaming your problems on a challenging childhood, you've bucked up and tried to see things from their point of view, forgive them for what they didn't know, or see the spiritual reason for it all. Or maybe you've found gratitude for the adversity that's made you the stronger, more resilient person you are today.

These coping mechanisms for dealing with adversity are valid. But this shellac of blue is not the true blue I'm talking about. "Taking the high road" or being in the faux blue is avoiding pain that needs to be felt in order to get to the deep ocean of blue. I don't mean to suggest you're not happy in your life, or that your resilience and accomplishments are any less meaningful. I'm suggesting that our minds can make sophisticated rationalizations and create narratives that sound great, but our body will tell another story until we get real about the red.

If you are reading this thinking you do a pretty good job at being in the blue, notice how far that blue lands in your system. Be especially rigorous with yourself about staying with present moment blue, not the idea of it, but the felt sense experience of it. Blue happens in the body—it is an experience of what *is* pleasurable, not an idea of what should be pleasurable.

If you're someone who is stuck in the superficial blue, you might have noticed that your friends are sometimes confused or frustrated by your responses to difficult experiences or feelings. When they share their pain, you tend to offer advice that points to the larger context or a more positive outcome. You may also find yourself taking on way more responsibility for your part in relationships, believing that if you focus on what you can control, the relationship will improve. I love the idea of account-ability, but being mired in a false blue can create unrealistic ex-pectations, and a lot of unnecessary emotional labor that could be avoided by simply recognizing the red.

Chronic fake blue–finding can also provide justifications to stay in unhealthy or abusive relationships. Sometimes, leaving a situation is the only blue option. It's not escape, it's not failure, it's not taking the cowardly way—it's the only way. You cannot regulate your nervous system within an abusive or violent rela-tionship. There is no blue in abuse. Your body is feeling alarm for a reason. It's signaling you that there's an actual threat. These body security systems are in place for a reason.

THE UPPER LIMIT PROBLEM AND HOLD IT MOMENTS

I learned about the challenge of experiencing higher heights or more pleasure from *The Big Leap* written by Stanford professor and relationship coach Gay Hendricks. He describes how for a period of time he paid attention to all the conflicts and fights he was having with his wife. He started to realize that instead of being a sign of big problems, they all came after moments of huge intimacy, expansion, or connection. So he named these "upper limit" problems. His system would be stretched beyond its normal margins with the goodness, and then lo and behold in the days following there would be conflict. They would pendulate to a place of contraction and discord.

Hendricks explains that when he and his wife started seeing their conflicts not as a problem to be solved, or as evidence that there was something wrong in their relationship, but instead as their nervous systems responding to growth, everything shifted. They could then support and soothe each other. They could be more tender with each other as they realized the disappointment from or attachment to the wonderful experiences they'd had. Then they stopped fighting, almost altogether!

You might not be in a relationship, but upper limit problems can manifest in many different forms. Maybe you have a great date, but then spend a lot of time deciding that it probably wasn't as good as you thought, or they're not the right person for you, and you sabotage any potential with bad communication or no communication at all. Maybe you start an exercise routine and are feeling really good, and then you just peter off, and go back to your old routine that doesn't feel as good. Maybe you make more money than you have from a client, but then lose motivation to keep working. These are all signs of upper limit problems—our difficulty with rising to new thresholds, sustaining them, and growing capacity to be comfortable in a new normal without collapsing back into our familiar range.

For me the upper limit problem was the ultimate reframe. And it led me to a practice that has become a joke among my friends—we give each other a side-eye glance and playfully say, "Hoooold it." Holding it means staying with the celebratory moments, however small. If someone gives you a compliment, can you pause, take a breath, and instead of deflecting or batting the compliment away, can you take it in and hold it? Can you hold that sensation, without making sense of it, explaining it, making a compliment right back, or changing the subject? If your child gets an award or has a performance, can you allow yourself to beam with pride—to take it in, and to hold it? If you finish one project, can you let there be space inside you to feel that completion, rather than just moving right on to the next thing that has to be done? Can you look at that bigger number in your bank account, marvel at it, and let the good news settle all the way in?

There will always be a next thing. In the absence of a lot of formal ritual, it's even more important to give ourselves these mini punctuations. "Hold it" moments let all parts of ourselves sync up with a new reality, a new identity. If we rush through them or past them, we're more prone to experiencing those bigger backslides. Throughout this book, I want you to allow for these pauses and the acknowledgment of gains or insights you are making. Again and again, I see students making huge strides, like learning to name sensations in their body and daring to communicate them, reporting that gain, and then concluding with "I know it's no big deal, and I have a long way to go." These small changes *are* a big deal. We can tell ourselves that! And we can tell our friends that, too. Just that phrase: "That's a really big deal." It pauses the conversation and gives emphasis to growth and big experiences. We grow our capacity for goodness together.

Many of us have internalized the belief that pleasure is the reward we receive once we heal our trauma. Once we fix this or that thing, once we get this job or that boyfriend, then we'll feel good or trust enough to allow ourselves to relax and enjoy ourselves. We're constantly finding reasons to delay feeling good, or saving up feeling good for weekends or vacation. Even our self-care or spiritual practices can take a serious "should" tone. We treat pleasure as something that we have to earn, from working hard and paying dues. We see it as separate from us rather than a part of us.

This is not how the nervous system functions—in order to grow we must start in blue. We cannot heal trauma without the ability to feel pleasure. We need a reference point and a foothold in our body, and specifically what feels good in our body. Pleasure has to be part of the journey, not just the imagined destination. Pleasure is not out there waiting to be discovered. Pleasure is in here, waiting to be discovered right now and along the way. Experiment with saying, "I'm here and I'm alive." Take all the time you can to let that soak in.

You're here and you're alive.

We're here and we're alive.

CHAPTER 5

UNDERSTAND THE PREDATOR-PREY DYNAMIC

A common reason that it's difficult for people to land or orient to pleasure, or "blue" as we're calling it, is because so many people feel numb, frozen, or totally out of touch with their bodies. If the body hasn't been a safe place to be in the past, we may have learned to live mostly in the world of thoughts, intellect, or imagination, and that affects our ability to have a relationship to our body in the present moment. There's nowhere to land blue. So we need to call all the parts of ourselves home, by pausing, taking time to let our body speak and learn its language, and then soaking and shaking loose some of the sediment of those past experiences.

Thus far you've developed a deeper sense of where you are in space, a sense of what's yours and not yours—what belongs to you and what doesn't—and a nuanced way to track your internal experience. All these skills and principles are the foundation for doing reparative work. Healing can happen through coming out of "freeze," or moving out of being stuck in one sympathetic response, and restoring different responses to your nervous system.

Freeze can look different depending on the individual. For some, it may manifest physically as coldness in the body, particularly in the hands and feet. For others it might appear as a general sense of disconnection, lack of vitality, or unreachability. If you default to freeze, you may find yourself often in a haze, unable to make decisions, not knowing where to go, or feeling stuck. You may experience your general rhythm as slow—from your heart rate to your blood pressure to your pace of conversations. You might procrastinate a lot and find it hard to locate your own genuine energy or drive. You might find yourself listening a lot more than talking, or unable to keep up with others in conversations. Or you might literally freeze—lose your words, get stuck in your seat, or find yourself in a thousand-mile stare.

Some of these examples are low-level freeze tendencies that aren't necessarily harmful on a larger scale—you can just wear warm socks if your feet are cold—but they may be useful to help you understand how these tendencies are rooted in your physiological responses to perceived danger or threat. When we start to listen, feel, and identify the incomplete stress responses that live underneath freeze, we can eventually thaw out and free up energy so we can play and be available to pleasure.

As we begin this work, I want you to keep in mind that the foundational principle is loving-kindness toward ourselves for however we have reacted in the past, and whatever has carried over into the present. These are not cognitive decisions; they are physiological outcomes. Hopefully knowing that there is nothing "wrong" with you, and that your body has made its best effort to keep you safe in the past, will help you build an ever-deepening reservoir of radical self-acceptance. That's the undercurrent that I want us to return to and fortify as we go.

Take a moment now to acknowledge one thing that you appreciate about yourself. Maybe it's the courage that you have to keep looking at yourself, maybe it's the devotion you have to understanding the nature of things, maybe it's how much you care for your clients or children or partner. Pick one thing. Let it sink in. Make a statement out of it. "I am brave in my willingness to work on myself." "I am kind to others." "I really want to be of service." Allow that statement to permeate you, like a drop of food coloring in water. Stay with the feeling-tone of the statement for a minute or so. Close your eyes for a moment, so that you can really be with it. Of course, the pendulation will happen, your system will present you with the red—that you aren't brave enough, or that you secretly resent someone, or that you aren't doing enough to help. Ignore that pendulation and self-questioning and return to the statement again. Allow for blue sensations, emotions, or movement to appear in your awareness.

As you go through this process of letting your body speak, many new things will start to happen that may feel strange. You might find that your body moves itself—swaying, yawning, twisting, shaking, or turning. You may find yourself making sounds—sighing, humming, groaning, even burping. These movements and sounds, in this context also called *discharge*, are your body's way of releasing stored energy from the movements and sounds it could not make in the past, and completing them, or smoothing those record skips.

Each culture has its own social pressure about the ways we should behave and compose ourselves that are acceptable. Without such rules and norms, these movements and sounds would occur naturally, leaving us with less stored-up emotion, tension, and residue. You may start to notice some of these movements happen spontaneously as you start to live in the world through your felt sense, which becomes more available the more responsive we are.

Freezing is self-protective, and often highly effective; however, it leaves our bodies with unexpressed sympathetic responses, movements that could not be made in the moment. We weren't able to say what we needed to say or do what we needed to do. Those words, gestures, and actions are stored in the nervous system. When we default to freeze patterning, we aren't able to defend ourselves actively against a present threat. In order to fully recover from a freeze experience—whether caused by anesthesia from surgery, feeling cornered by a dominating authority figure, daily racist microaggressions, being the victim of abuse or assault, or a combination of many things—we have to spiral up out of the parasympathetic freeze and into our fight-or-flight responses. We have to give the body its chance to speak, or move, or shake. We draw this understanding from observing the behavior of wild animals.

WILD ANIMALS DON'T EXPERIENCE TRAUMA

Here's how the predator-prey dynamic works in the wild, from a nervous system perspective.

A wolf hunts a rabbit. The wolf, salivating and pacing, starts its careful approach, getting closer and closer. At some point, the rabbit senses that it is being stalked, stops moving (freezes), and scans the environment, staying as still as possible in hopes that the wolf won't see it and continue approaching. If the wolf does continue its zigzag approach, the rabbit will "play dead" (collapse). The words "play dead" make it sound like it decided to collapse, but in fact, its system shut down. Then if the wolf is still interested, it will come pick up the rabbit by the neck and shake it around to confirm if the rabbit is dead or not. Predators don't usually want dead prey. If the wolf is convinced the rabbit is dead, it will simply drop it and run off. When the rabbit senses that the wolf is gone, it opens its eyes to look around (visual orientation), and its little ears perk up and flash back and forth (auditory orientation). If, through its senses, the rabbit perceives safety, it will bolt upright to all fours, continuing to look around in the environment. Next the rabbit shakes, and continues shaking until a seemingly spontaneous ending when the shaking subsides and the rabbit runs off. The cycle is complete. The rabbit doesn't hop around trembling for the rest of the day and avoiding the pasture. The wolf doesn't stalk that same area again and again. They go on without the imprint of that hunt impeding or determining how they behave in the future.

In Somatic Experiencing school, we watch videos of some of these scenes. The first time I watched one, I was on the edge of my seat, grimacing, cheering for the rabbit, gripped, just hoping with all my might that it would escape. Afterward, the teacher asked us who identified with the rabbit and who identified with the wolf. In my mind, everyone identified with the rabbit—who doesn't cheer for the underdog? To my surprise, about 30 percent of the students identified with the wolf. They reported that they were salivating and excited. The other 70 percent, like me, were tense and a little scared.

In that moment, I had a reckoning. I couldn't characterize the predator instinct as "bad" and "wrong" and the "enemy," because the people who identified with the predator role were people that I actually knew, liked, and thought of as "good" people. In that moment, I also understood that everything from the kinds of movies I like (against-all-odds success stories) to many of my major life choices (becoming a vegetarian, advocating for social justice) were fueled by my overidentification with the prey side of the nervous system. You might read this and think these are all "good" choices—and they could be, if they are actually conscious, considered choices—but if they are default options dictated by my stressed physiological response, then they indicate a nervous system default.

I've worked with women who assist refugee populations, treat critically injured patients in the ER, attend rape crisis hotlines, or otherwise serve on the frontlines of helping others. Their dedication is notable, but oftentimes what we perceive as a nobility or strength of character is in fact the product of trauma; they are drawn to dangerous situations because that's what their nervous system recognizes as familiar. Healing from trauma offers us the ability and opportunity to reevaluate what healthy environments look like for us, to identify environments where we can regulate ourselves without being exposed to a continuous level of stress, in the exact spots where we may need our own healing. Many of my clients became sick before they realized that they were retraumatizing themselves with their diet or their work. Their body set the limit for them.

The reason wild animals don't experience trauma, but humans and domesticated animals do, is because humans are not always able to complete the cycle in the way we saw the rabbit behave earlier. Wild animals experience all kinds of hardships, struggles, and profoundly shocking life-altering events in their lives, but they don't experience those events as traumas once they are over. Without a way to move through the complete nervous system cascade, these same events often live on as trauma in humans and pets.

Our systems get interrupted in different places along this cycle of what we call activation (stress response) and deactivation or discharge. Have you ever tripped on a rough edge of sidewalk and then just kept walking along as if nothing happened because acknowledging it would be socially embarrassing? Many things can interrupt the completion of cycles—social norms and self-consciousness, surgery and anesthesia, and betrayals and boundary ruptures.

Remember, when we are not under threat, our sympathetic nervous system drives us to move and act. Our parasympathetic nervous system lets us rest, digest, and slow down. Our sympathetic nervous system is the accelerator; our parasympathetic nervous system is the brake. We need a toned autonomic nervous system that's working in cyclical coordination so that we have cycles of activity and rest, eating and elimination, arousal and orgasm.

Generally speaking in our society, a sympathetic nervous system reaction has been acceptable for men, both the healthy and unhealthy aspects. Everything from assertive, domineering, and dominant behavior to expressions of anger or violence is allowed or even expected—and therefore those circuits are well-worn. For women, it's just the opposite: we are expected to express a sympathetic flight reaction in response to stress—fear or panic—or the parasympathetic response to stress— collapsing or crying—or the freeze response of stoicism. In other words, it's been more socially acceptable for men to be wolves, or predators, and for women to be rabbits, or prey. This doesn't map onto all situations at all times, but it is a common power dynamic. We know that these reactions are the result of both biological imperative and social conditioning. Unfortunately, though, we have assigned moral value to these responses—categorizing the predator role as "bad," and the prey role as "good"—when in reality both responses can be highly adaptive (the rabbit got away from the wolf, after all).

Sometimes I work with women who are dealing with "freeze" issues as a result of having literally been trapped in situations— maybe they were physically overpowered, or perhaps medicated, like during birth or a surgery. Whatever the cause, their body was forced into a state of immobility at the time. When we are able to go back into the implicit memory of the body with the resources we have developed together, their bodies will often make the movements that could not be made at the time.

For example, when Liza came to see me, she was dealing with chronic pelvic and inner thigh pain. She shared that while she was in labor, she was afraid that her doctor was going to do something that she did not agree to, and she was particularly terrified of an episiotomy. She was squeezing her legs together as tightly as she could, which in retrospect she realized was delaying labor quite a bit, because her body was tightening rather than opening for the baby to come out. During our session, we talked about the kind nurse who kept looking into her eyes and telling her it was okay to soften (blue). Then she pendulated to red, recalling a deep distrust and fear of being injured, tears falling down her cheeks. Shortly after, her right leg started to tremble, and she realized that at the time she'd had an urge to kick her doctor (fight response). She never would have done it at that moment in the past, but her body was holding on to the impulse. She needed the opportunity to move that leg and complete that innate response to fight the doctor, who was registering to her as a threat. So in the here and now, she pressed her leg as if kicking against my hand while I gave her a bit of resistance. Her body was finally able to do what it could not do when under threat—execute an instinctual self-protective movement. Liza's pelvic pain resolved shortly after this work. She had done some physical therapy and movement therapy trying to release and strengthen the muscles, but until we got to the underlying nervous system pattern, she did not experience true relief.

These connections may seem miraculous and overly simplified when we are used to working from a top-down psychological model. That approach might have us questioning why: "Why were you afraid of an episiotomy?" "Why was the doctor threatening?" Or a more emotional approach: "How did that make you feel?" or "What did that remind you of?"

The bottom-up approach applies curiosity to the question

"what?"—"What is happening right now in the body?" "When you say these words, what happens in the body?" or "When I think this thought, what sensations or emotions do I notice in my body?" The truth is that our bodies are incredibly responsive and right there waiting for the attuned listener that speaks its language. That listener might be a skilled somatic practitioner. But we can also become fluent in the language of our own bodies, able to parse out the different sounds and signals. Then the body doesn't need to shout to get our attention. We hear the earlier whispers and can act on them. We are learning a language that is more primitive and foundational than our spoken language.

Before we invite in these bigger situations for renegotiation, we first have to create a safe context where we can begin to thaw the parts of ourselves that have been in freeze. We often experience freeze in the center of the body—our guts and organs. Digestive issues, from constipation to irritable bowel system, are related to ongoing freeze responses. As you come out of freeze and mobilize freeze responses, you might notice more sensations in your pelvis, belly, or chest.

We will begin by making sound from low down into the pelvis and belly. Making sound is already one step into action. The next step is feeling the vibration of this sound in the belly, starting to shake loose some of the sediment. And then using TIMES, you can track what else happens in your system as a result of waking up some dormant places.

"VU" PRACTICE

Take a moment to feel yourself in your seat wherever you are and to retract your gaze away from the book or the screen so that you can bring your focus inside a bit more. We know from past chapters that we can orient to the external environment and we can also orient to our internal environment—toggling back and forth from our inner world to our outer world. A healthy nervous system can move in and out and back in and back out without the loss of one world in favor of the other. So when we orient out, we don't lose ourselves; we can still have a sense of who we are. As we orient in, we can still be located in and be aware of our surroundings.

Notice your foundation, and make yourself as comfortable as possible. Check in with your breath. We're going to make the sound "vu" together, v-u. You may have taken a yoga class before and chanted the sound "om." It's just like that except we use the sound "vu." The sound "vu" reverberates in the enteric nervous system—in the guts—so that's why we use it.

Allow for a normal exhale, and then a full inhale. On the next exhale, letting the air and sound come from as deep down in your torso as possible, make the sound "vu" at as low of a tone as possible without strain. Allow that sound to resonate as deep down as you can. You might feel it in your chest or your belly and organs or your womb space or all the way down into your pelvis and vagina. Draw it out until there's no more breath, and then just let your breath be free. Pause in the silence to hear and feel the inner sounds. In this experiment, the pause is just as important as the sound-making itself.

Notice on a sensation level what happens for you now during the pause. You might feel some heat, you might feel some gentle rocking, you might feel some pulsation in your hands or your arms or feet. Allow for that wave to go all the way through. If you don't feel much, no big deal.

One more time, make the sound of "vu," if you want to; if you don't want to, you don't have to do it.

Again, we are just noticing what comes up. And if you feel compelled to move in the pause, do so slowly, and as you're doing those movements, be present with them, throughout their whole range. Sometimes we just get habitual and start stretching or cracking our neck or moving in all these known ways that are not helping us stay with what's happening in the moment. We're just defaulting into the well-worn grooves, instead of going more slowly to see what's just underneath that habit, and potentially establishing a new groove. Moving your body is different from being moved by your body. If you move your body, go slowly enough that you're able to notice what's happening inside as you're doing it. That probably means moving at about 25 percent of the speed that you would normally go.

You may feel some spontaneous movement, very different from stretching. Allow your body to move you. If you feel like your head is moving itself without you moving it intentionally, then it's possible you're experiencing a motor response that at some time in the past wasn't complete. It's a very different sensation from cracking your neck or pulling it from side to side. We want to encourage and allow for the involuntary, nonhabitual movements to complete themselves.

If you're still on board, and it feels enlivening to make these sounds, we're going to layer in some deliberate movements. This time we're going to "vu," and as we do, you're going to open and close your mouth and lips like a guppy as you make this sound. The sound of "vu" will change as the shape of your mouth is changing. It will sound more like "vu-aaaah-vu-aaaah." If you're not feeling the sound resonate at all, you might want to put your hands on your lower belly.

When you're done with the sound and the slow opening and closing of your mouth, notice heat or coolness, streaming or stillness, upward or downward, any gentle rocking, and if you are rocking, just notice what could be comforting about that. Yawning is parasympathetic downregulation. Some people start to yawn a lot as their system regulates itself and unwinds. There's no right or wrong response. We're developing the ability to sense our bodies as we introduce some activation to slowly melt freeze responses.

Now we're going to do the same thing, "vu" with movement of the mouth, but instead of moving your lips, we're going to do it back at the jaw. Don't stretch your jaw as wide as it will go. Just make a relatively small movement, and notice you're not just moving your lips now, you're moving from your temporomandibular joint, your jaw back by your ear.

Notice in the pause, if a big breath follows, or if you are salivating more, what happens in the lungs and the muscles of your spine. You might notice some of these sensations or other ones I haven't named. There's no limit to the variety of sensations. You might like some of them more than others. You might not feel much at all. See if you can ride the wave of activation and deactivation. We are accustomed to feeling charge (which right now is the "vu" sound and movements we are making) and then just continuing on, without pausing to really notice the wave of activation rise and the wave of deactivation fall. We need the wave to come all the way back down—a feeling analogous to throwing a pebble in a lake, watching the ripples until there are no more left, and the lake is still again. That's the moment to throw another pebble, or in this case, make another sound.

Now we're layering in movements. We're going to use our hands, and you're going to mimic what you're doing with your mouth and your hands at the same time. So just adding on, and you can always go back a step if this is getting too much for you. You know it's too much if you're starting to think about a lot of other things, or you are wanting it to be over. If that's the case, then pause and orient yourself. You can even tell yourself your name and what you're doing, either silently to yourself or out loud.

Bring your hands up in front of you as if you were gesturing "hold on." The palms of your hands will be at chest-level facing forward with your elbows softly bent. It should feel comfortable. After a deeper inhale, make the sound "vu" as you open and close your mouth, within a reasonable range (we're not going for a major jaw stretch), and now open and close your hands as you open and close your mouth. Match the opening and closing of your mouth with the opening and closing of your hands.

Just notice again in the pause: Do you feel more energy in your system? Do you feel less energy in your system? Have emotions or images arisen? It's tempting to try to make meaning of the experience before you even have an experience, so instead let's see if we can just come back to the movement, sensation, or emotion channel. See if you can notice the temptation to jump up to the mind and coax yourself back into your bodily experience.

You may notice there are some sensations in your arms or your feet. When there's sympathetic discharge, it often expresses through the limbs because we use our arms and legs to fight or flee. We need to move our feet to get away or block our face or body with our arms to push someone away. So if you notice streaming sensations or tingling or anything like that in your arms and legs, just stay present with it until it settles back out. That can take different lengths of time, so be patient with it. Wait until it feels like the sensations have dissipated all the way.

We're introducing activation into the system by making sound with movements. For each movement, each person, and each day, it will take a different length of time for full deactivation to take place. We want to allow for enough time to come all the way down the back side of the wave. The bigger the input, stimulus, or event, the more time and space it may take for the charge to dissipate. Riding out the full cycle of the wave allows us to release tension and stress that have nothing to do with our present reality. Riding all the way down the back side of the wave is what allows contractions during birth, which themselves are waves, to remain manageable. If we carry charge from one contraction to the next, without being able to soften, relax, and let go in the intervals, the next contraction will register to our system as much stronger and more painful.

These waves are also a part of sexual arousal. If we don't allow for pauses, then we just keep ramping up the activation. Eventually our system won't be able to tolerate it and will need to discharge or offload, which can result in climaxing before we've had a chance to experience full arousal. Oftentimes this means we end up at the same destination over and over again, which can feel more like stress relief than generative, life-enhancing energy. On the other hand, if we observe the pauses, settle into them, breathe inside them, our arousal energy, or charge, can continue to build, and we will be able to move into a new level of capacity for activation, pleasure, and orgasmic possibility.

OWNING YOUR EXPERIENCE COMES BEFORE FORGIVENESS

Many of you may be highly identified with the prey role, like I've been, both in your nervous system and the way that you have constructed personality, behaviors, and worldview. If so, remember that there are many "blues" in this orientation. You care deeply about other sentient beings. You want to do what's right, not just for you, but for everyone. You don't think resources are there for the taking. These are all wonderful intentions. The world needs your empathy and deep concern. However, this nervous system propensity can be tricky and sometimes harmful for you, as your self-protective responses are disarmed when you direct your care outward rather than inward. There also may be a deeper learned helplessness that is prohibiting you from accessing and perceiving the raw true power that lives in your animal body and is there for you to claim and inhabit.

You may notice yourself skipping to gratitude, forgiveness, or seeing the point of view of the other person before you let the pain and anger register for yourself, before you even know where you stand. Maybe you feel it's really unfair to be quarantined alone with a newborn, for example, but any time anger about your situation rises up, you suppress it by thinking about how many others have it worse. Or you're grieving the cancer diagnosis of a friend, but that seems insignificant in light of the losses others have experienced, so you push yourself to get over it. Or you feel you have no right to feel overwhelmed, because you have White privilege, so you should just be quiet and use it.

Few of us want to be viewed as a victim or as having a "victim mentality," so we develop socially acceptable coping mechanisms. This could look like "seeing the best in someone," "being fair," "being the bigger person," or "taking the high road." Spiritual bypassing or skipping to a spiritual rationale is a common way to sidestep trauma and the difficult feelings and sensations that arise from personal, relational, and systemic conflicts. Those stances help keep prevailing family dynamics and social dynamics intact, especially when they're used to rationalize or explain away other people's bad behavior. This might look like anything from creepy behavior to codependence to mental or physical abuse to racism. So many kinds of bad behaviors are left unaddressed because of these freezes in the nervous system.

Yet the mental steps toward the high road are precipitous if we haven't let the gravity of the boundary infraction fully register. There's no denying it's painful to confront the ways that we may have taken on the prey role. But it's more painful to mask the truth and impact those situations have had on us, that live on in our body. We are afraid of the depth of suffering that is there.

We want to come to a place of resolution and "get over it." Yet, in this process, the body is left out of these choices. Your mind might have forgiven, but your body has not.

When you skip the sympathetic step of acknowledging your anger (fight) or sadness (flight) or the parasympathetic response of hopelessness, then you end up in faux blue—seeing the lessons and going over the top in taking responsibility for parts in a dynamic that are not yours. You overcompensate for what you see as wrong with the world, and in turn end up weakened, with less of a sense of your own power and efficacy, or with disease in your body. To restore a sense of power does not mean to give up your values of equality. It may feel selfish, at first, but as you slowly come out of freeze, over time, you will feel the truth and power in your own body. You will know how to contain your energy and have more traction toward your purpose and your life. It will become obvious where you can be effective, what's yours to take care of and what is not.

You may also identify with having predator energy in certain situations and prey energy in others. For instance, you might be very assertive at work, but less in command when it comes to relationships. Or you might even feel like you're stuck in predator mode and aren't easily able to access prey mode. But I can assure you that all of us have the capacity to occupy the full range of our nervous systems—the full range of human, mammalian experience—from full dominance to total submission. I think it's worth remembering here again that "predator" is not good or bad, and "prey" is not good or bad. They are functions. The health of the rabbit population is in part governed by the wolf. The health of the wolves relies in no small part with the rabbit . . . to name only two in this web. They have an interdependent relationship. They are far ends of one kind of pendulation. As humans, we get to occupy the full spectrum.

CHAPTER 6

ACTIVATE YOUR INNER PREDATOR

Now that we've worked on thawing what's frozen, the next step toward healing is to direct our attention to the process of restoring the predator side of the nervous system.

My hope is that by now it doesn't feel as scary to embrace your predator side because you know that this isn't about becoming hyperassertive or becoming an "alpha female." It's not about becoming domineering or disrespectful, although it might feel that way at first if you've never exercised this part of your system. All of those posturings—from domineering to disrespectful—are overcompensations. Restoring the predator side of our system is about coming into contact with our natural impulses of self-protection and self-defense, trusting that those will kick in if and when we need them. It's about getting out of freeze in order to create something new, so that your default response to threat doesn't have to be prey.

Ultimately our goal is to establish a wider net of support beneath us that's just ours. Many times we question our inner radar and wonder if a situation is actually unsafe or if we just *feel* unsafe. But when we do this work, we can develop a reliable radar.

We can develop confidence. We can learn to defend ourselves, care for ourselves, leave an unsafe situation. In other words, our need to protect and hold on to ourselves becomes greater than our concerns about making too much noise, being nice, disappointing someone, or being a "bad patient," "bad daughter," "needy girl-friend," or whatever role you may feel compelled to fill. This ferocity is an embodiment of self-love and unquestioned self-worth.

Imagine this scene: A couple is in bed. They start kissing, and it's getting hot. The man starts to climb on top of his wife and just as he moves his second leg, she starts to clam up. They both feel it—her past trauma rising to "ruin" the moment. But this time, as she feels the freeze coming on, she names it. "I don't want to go here again, I'm starting to freeze, I'm starting to get emotional. I have to get up." So they get out of bed, and they face each other. She's been taking my classes, so she decides to try something different. She starts to bounce around, working out the freeze, and eventually makes some "ooooh" and "vuuuu" and "grrrrr" sounds. The man thinks, "Why not?" and joins in. Now they're both jumping up and down, making noises, and then laughing with each other. They move around for fifteen or twenty minutes staying connected. They feel a little absurd, and a little embarrassed, but soon they both feel victorious. They didn't return to bed to have sex that night. But they didn't fall into the familiar trap either. Something different happened, creating more safety, connection, and truth to what was honest in that moment—a need to move out of the flight and freeze prey response and into action, and they did it together.

When the woman opted to stand up and change positions, she got herself out of freeze by engaging the healthy sympathetic nervous system. She made a new choice, moving away from the emotion channel into the movement channel. She was in control, and an active director of the experience—opposite to the freeze that paralyzed her when she experienced trauma. Her mind knows this partner is safe, but her nervous system is registering him, and sex, as unsafe based on past experience. Rather than defaulting all the way into the parasympathetic freeze mode, she gave her sympathetic nervous system the space to act, to do what she needed to do to help her feel safe and connected—she is no longer stuck in the prey response.

Embodying your inner predator isn't just about gaining a sense of power in the bedroom; it impacts all of your life. It can help you set boundaries as a parent, gain confidence at work, and embrace your privilege so that your response to injustice is more meaningful and productive. If you are not in a privileged body, embracing your predator role can help you mobilize your grief, shock, or fear so that you can feel comfortable taking up space and letting yourself be heard. Ultimately it's about giving yourself a sense of irrevocable safety, because you know you can protect or defend yourself at any time. You also know that you probably won't need to.

If you're thinking, "I could never do that"—believe me, you can, and as silly or timid as you may feel at first, as you progress through this work it feels absolutely amazing. I know because embracing the predator was a central part of my healing. I began my journey while living in Brazil. At that time, I realized that after being in therapy on and off for over fifteen years, I had only ever worked with women. Somehow I knew I would only be able to go so far working with female therapists because I wasn't threatened by women the way I was by men. This hadn't stopped me from having male friends, boyfriends, and a marriage, but there was something deeper that I was trying to uncover. I wanted to create a deeper level of safety and understanding with men.

I chose a male somatic therapist who was a martial artist, ballroom dancer, and yoga teacher and happened to be from the

Amazon. I had already begun my own somatic therapy studies, or what I affectionately call "trauma school." When I showed up for my first session and told him that I wanted to work on boundaries with men, I cried for the rest of the session. I didn't narrate anything about my history; simply being in his male presence and acknowledging this vulnerability began to have an impact on my system.

I trusted that the work would be helpful, even though it felt confusing. My mind thought I was further along in my healing than my body and emotions suggested at that moment. Slowly over the course of several sessions, he began to escalate aggressive gestures and behaviors toward me, allowing me to reorganize my body and my nervous system in response and to find my literal ground. He began to stalk me, then he would physically lunge at me, and eventually we would wrestle and spar. One day he called me an *onça*, or jaguar, because of my freckles and golden-colored skin, and it was through this process with him that I claimed my place in the role of jaguar. I no longer needed to identify as victim or survivor. Occasionally words, thoughts, or images would arise that related to a past sexual assault or a relationship I had with a guru. I never told him all the stories of what had happened to me or deconstructed the "why" of all the alarm and emotions that would come up. I developed confidence in my ability to stay alert, not freeze, and defend myself when necessary. I could trust my internal radar.

I had already tried so many kinds of therapy—EMDR (eye movement desensitization and reprocessing); Enneagram-informed, Jungian depth psychology; not to mention that I was an experienced, well-trained yoga teacher and bodyworker myself—yet nothing was as effective for me as this somatic therapy. I'll never know if the earlier support I gained primed my system to be ready to do this final piece of work, or if the earlier therapies simply made me feel like I was doing something, when actually I was reinforcing some of the patterns by talking so much about them. I think it's probably a combination of both. I forged some very special relationships with the therapists who walked with me through dark times; their presence was a deep comfort and offered healthy attachment when I needed it. But the first time I endeavored Somatic Experiencing, every cell in my body knew this work was going to be different. I was in awe and disbelief that in all the years of dancing, yoga practice, and therapy, I hadn't touched on this deceptively simple tool.

Over time, my traumatic experiences didn't feel as significant and rarely impacted my sexuality. Now, I rarely think about the specific events. The word "rape" doesn't make me wince and flashback. I can hear stories of many women and not fall into the dark pit of my own trauma. I share the details of my past now only when it is significant to light the way for others to come along through this maze.

One of the regular corners of the maze where I got turned around and stuck was with parenting. Studying and embodying my inner predator showed me patterns of healthy aggression and dominance that I realized my daughter needed me to display for her own safety and maturation. I'd been avoiding those behaviors with my rational expressions of democracy and mutual respect. But, in fact, she was dominating me, without me even realizing I'd given away all my power. I was talking her through situations, explaining everything, when what she also needed was physical engagement demonstrating *embodiment* of healthy dominance and hierarchy—nonverbally communicating to her that I was in charge. I would do so in cycles—training her system that there is a space in any cycle for rest and that you don't just keep winding and winding and winding yourself up. Like we've been doing together in the practices in this book, there's a period of activation and then you pause, absorb, and integrate before starting a new cycle. Through this practice we developed a new vocabulary that allowed her to relax and feel her place in the order of things—a child with a parent who will contain and protect her. There is no question about who's in charge.

This healing and empowerment is possible for you, too. You can reclaim the predator and activate your inner jaguar. Your past imprints will not be released, but their hold on you will. You can learn to coordinate your facial expressions, the content of your words, your vocal tone, and your spinal posture so that yeses and nos are nonnegotiable. You can untangle the crossed wires of what you are communicating with your nervous system so that when you say no, your children stop climbing on you the first time you ask. You will learn to start saying yes with your eyes, your words, and your body to create an opening to invite attention you do want. You can ask for a raise without backpedaling. You can decline an invitation to the PTA meeting without equivocating, apologizing, or offering something else you don't have time to offer. You can stand in your true desires.

FROM FAWNING TO FEROCITY

A while back, one of my friends asked me to roar as she took a picture of me. When I saw the image, I was shocked; I looked like a kid pretending to be fierce. I didn't look angry or scary or intimidating at all. My default nervous system response in the sympathetic branch is usually flight (worry and fear). So my face often reflects that worry. I've joked that I was born with a furrowed brow: inquisitive, serious, and a little worried—the default facial expression I mentioned in chapter 3. I usually feel afraid or sad before I feel angry, and my inability to mobilize anger and show it was reflected in the picture.

That misalignment of verbal and physical expressions has also been modeled to me by many of my clients, who will use a forceful word like "stop" but then laugh right afterward, or cock their head to one side, or avert their eyes as they say it. Their sounds and movements diminished the power of their words. Their niceness—in part, a social nervous system response—was visible on their face in permanent smiles or head tilts of deference. These types of gestures indicate the need to maintain social rapport—a habit that, in turn, overrode their self-protective instincts. As we've discussed, as a culture we've not permitted women to show sympathetic fight responses, and as a result, we are often not well-practiced in them. What that means is that we don't always look angry when we are angry. That's a problem.

In the process of writing this book, I shared my jaguar process with a prominent neuroscientist, curious to see if she would draw any parallels between what I was seeing in my work with the body and what she knew from her work with the brain. She immediately responded that it was a bad idea to teach women how to look angry or scornful or disgusted. Their likability, she said, goes way down—it puts women at a disadvantage professionally and socially. While I was frustrated by her response, in a way, she actually proved my point. As women, we know it's a problem for other people when we show anger. That's precisely why we've learned so well how to be nice, how to build bridges, how to see a situation from other people's points of view, and how to mask our genuine impulses. And in turn, we've scrambled our self-protective responses.

Mobilizing facial muscles related to the fight response that have been underused or dormant is an inside-out way of restoring our sympathetic responses. Imagine a rabbit's nose twitching quickly as it sniffs around a meadow—those muscles that are very close to the side bridges of the nose. I had a client who experienced a similar twitching every time she would go on a long drive with her abusive husband. She never understood why it was happening—but it is clear to me that her body was reacting to the threat it felt and expressing fear through that mini-movement. At the time she didn't consciously realize she was feeling threatened, but her body was displaying the fear it felt. Once she was out of the marriage, she noticed that several bodily habits, like the rabbit nose scrunching and frequent urination, went away.

For a moment, right now, let's channel your predator and show your fangs—lifting your upper lip right above your incisors, or canine teeth. You can lift one side at a time, Billy Idol style, or both upper lips at once. Bare your teeth. Of course, most of us will feel silly doing this. Unless you're an actor or a model, or maybe a selfie aficionado, you probably haven't spent a lot of time deliberately experimenting with facial expressions, especially ones that you might think are ugly. One of my students who learned to bare her teeth tried it with her dog. Instead of talking, shouting, or gesturing to get him to follow her commands, she looked at him and bared a canine tooth on one side. Her dog immediately calmed down and obeyed her. She thought it might be a fluke or that it would only work the first time, but it turns out that it's worked every single time she's needed her dog to stop barking or jumping up on her.

Of course, we're not going to walk around the world baring our teeth. These processes are all about developing the nervous system capacity in the full spectrum from predator to prey, so that our system has access to the appropriate responses when needed, which enables it to become more accurate and refined in its perception of threat. Mobilizing facial muscles we rarely use helps them come out of freeze—we're waking them up—and may allow for other parts of us to come out of freeze along with them. This outcome is similar to what takes place in our practice of TIMES—input into one channel can begin to mobilize or activate other channels, and that jostling can offer a new doorway to information we may not have had access to otherwise.

For instance, when you start to show your fangs, you might notice frustration (emotion—low-level sympathetic activation). That frustration might lead to tears (parasympathetic release) or a questioning of the exercise (sympathetic fight) or a desire to quit (parasympathetic resignation). Or you might start to laugh, and enjoy the absurdity of pretending to be an animal. You might want to share it with someone in play (social nervous system). You might resist this playfulness as a waste of time, and want to get to the "real work" remaining in evaluation (top down) of the exercise rather than the experiencing of it (bottom up). All of these reactions and experiences, and any I haven't named, are part of the process of restoring access to the full range of our nervous systems. I encourage you to stay curious and allow yourself to be surprised when unexpected impulses arise.

LEARNING HOW TO ROAR

In chapter 5, we worked with the sound "vu." We wanted to hit as low of a note as possible without pinning our chin to our throat or creating strain, and we wanted the sound to come from deep within us, as close to our pelvic and belly organs as possible. There is a big difference between a shrill scream, which happens in the throat, and a deep guttural roar.

I have always thought of myself as an uninhibited person. I laugh loudly and often. I'm not afraid to sing along to a song or dance in public, or twirl down an empty grocery aisle. So I was surprised when I was giving birth to my daughter, laboring in my apartment, that my mind trailed off wondering if my neighbors could hear the noises I was making. Was I being too loud? This was reminiscent of a nonconsensual sexual experience I had, where the thought of screaming for help crossed my mind, but I didn't, because the next thought was that I didn't want the other students in the dorm to hear me because then they would see me in this compromised sexual position. My system overrode my self-protective fight instincts in favor of its social nervous system circuitry.

Learning how to roar means learning how to deal with the surprise and sometimes unpredictability of what sound comes out, as well as how to take up space and how to be unapologetic. It flies in the face of being polite. Even if we don't consider ourselves people-pleasers or particularly well-mannered, in the face of threat, many of us do default to the social nervous system response of appeasement and proximity. We can practice growling and roaring. We'll layer on growling to the progression of the sound of "vu" along with hand movements.

Take a moment to allow your eyes to look around your space. Make sure to look behind you as well. Visually take in the whole space that you are in, slowly looking up and down. This process of visual orientation might take you a minute or so. There may be places that you look, where you notice a bigger breath, or a yawn, or a micromovement happen. Give orientation its own time. Place your hands on your low belly, and on an exhale let out the sound of "vu." Then add the opening and closing of the mouth together with opening and closing your hands. If you need to, go back to pages 111 to 116 and follow the more detailed description, because we are building on that sequence now. Then after you've practiced the sequence, return to this page tomorrow. Remember the principle of titration—we are adding in a little bit at a time so that your system can adjust toward greater organization and integration, without getting pushed over a threshold.

On an exhale, as you make the sound of "vu" and open your mouth, it will start to transform into the sound "ah," and as you open and close your mouth, experiment with making it into a "rawr"—a roaring sound. As you make the roaring noise, make the movements with your face more dramatic (even if it feels weird, and it will). Combine the movement of the jaw opening and closing with the baring of your teeth. Try this a couple times, and remember to pause in between, so you can track what's happening. Are you hotter or colder? Are you trembling a bit? Are you enjoying it, your face smiling or laughing? Ride that wave all the way through, before you start again for the next sound. You may want to do this in front of a mirror. When I teach this class online, because of the format, students can see themselves on the screen, and I can see them to give them tips. Looking at a mirror will allow you to see which parts of your face are moving and which aren't. Practice your ferocity making the roaring noise and baring your fangs. Let the sound come from as low in the torso as possible. Mean it.

If you only make the sound, or you only do the facial movements, that's a start. It's really the coordination of making a loud growl with the mobilization of the facial muscles where you will feel full power. So far, we only talked about facial movements from the nose down. Experiment with your eyes, your eyebrows, and your forehead. What is your truest expression of anger?

The fight response, when you move toward a threat, requires an activation of your flexor muscles. Your flexors are what make fists, curl your biceps, contract your frontal abdominal wall, and tuck your pelvis under. Your flexors also make the clawing action. So we are going to combine the sound, the jaw movement, the facial movement of baring the teeth, as well as a clawing action.

With your hands about your forearm's length in front of your chest, when you make the roaring sound, open and close your hands matching the pace of your mouth and hand movements. This time as you are closing your mouth, showing your fangs as if in a biting motion, add the clawing of your hands. You'll probably be able to do a few clawing/growling movements on one exhale. Your hands probably won't close all the way to fists. Feel your whole arms light up with this action. Get into it. Inhabit the feeling of the growling predator. Be intimidating and scary. Then pause. Track your system. Pause longer than you normally might be inclined to; stay with your inside experience. And when you've ridden that wave, let your eyes look around your space. Let them go where they want to go, as you toggle from inside awareness to outside awareness.

FULL BODY ACTIVATION

Find yourself some space on the ground where you can comfortably kneel down on all fours. From all fours, look around your space. Notice what's around you and especially behind you. Bring your hands a little closer to your knees than you would for a tabletop, so that your shoulders are an inch or two beyond your wrists. Then shift your weight forward and feel your shoulders go beyond your wrists, feel your haunches light up and get strong, and then rock back. Tuck your toes under as if you are on a sprinting starting block, and explore that felt sense of readiness, the energy from your legs all the way up through your arms, as you rock back and forth. Press through your feet as you incline forward, shifting your weight over through your activated clawing hands.

Look straight ahead and steady your gaze in front of you, at one target. Invite in the growling and roaring as you begin to crawl back and forth, side to side on all fours, maintaining your focus on that target, real or imaginary, in front of you. Go slowly and invite the predator energy inside of you. Become the jaguar. You are in pursuit. Maybe your elbows bend as you slink down toward the floor. Maybe you like to push your weight back toward your toes as you curl your tail under, ready to pounce. Maybe the sounds are a low rumble, maybe they're a full-bellied roar. Stick with the flexor energy, especially if you tend to be parasympathetic dominant. This can be weirdly exhausting, even if it doesn't feel like much. You also might feel energized. This could also change from round to round or day to day. When you get tired or bored, rest. Let it go. Track your system, look around. And then check in to see if you feel compelled to go for another round. If you're not sure, get up and walk around. Go to the bathroom, get a drink of water, shake it off a bit. After you've given your system time to deactivate, do you want to do another round? If you do, go for it. But remember, more isn't better. You can come back to this tomorrow or next week or any other time that feels right.

COMPLETING A LOOP

So far, we've explored the movements and sounds of a predator—to activate, mobilize, and coordinate patterns that may be totally new or underused or not completely in sync. We've done these exercises without deliberately bringing up any memories, but you may have had images or emotions or scenes return to you, without conjuring them. The movements and sounds themselves elicited the memories. Many women have experienced healing in this process without ever deliberately "working on" a specific trauma or event. They've found themselves feeling comfortable in a previously triggering situation without having intentionally focused on that situation during the course.

However, you might have had an experience or two—medical, or sexual, or otherwise—that led you to pick up this book. You may have put some pieces together, or remembered other situations connected to the ones you want to work on. Trauma repair offers the opportunity to complete unfinished cycles. I'll be honest: this is one of the most controversial parts of this book, and why it comes now, after you've created a foundation of orienting to the environment and coming home to yourself. Many therapists would balk at the prospect of someone trying to do trauma repair on their own, without the support of a skilled professional. Optimally we would all have access to skilled somatic professionals, and at the end of this book, you will find resources to help you find that support as well. In an ideal world, we would also have collective spaces of ritual that would encourage us to process this material in a safe community forum. But one thing I learned from the #MeToo movement was that the sheer volume of nervous system repair that's needed is massive—and I believe we have to attempt that reparative work from as many angles as we can. I've also been thrilled to witness my students, both in person and online, supercede my expectations for what I thought was possible in a group or virtual setting. The healing my students experienced gave me confidence that many women are ready and capable of making these repairs with the right tools and guidance that have usually been reserved to the domain of professionals. Remember these principles as we move forward. If you are starting to feel overwhelmed or a level of emotional reaction that's not manageable, orient to the present moment environment. Titration is key. Take the bite you can digest. You can pause or stop at any time. Nothing is mandatory to do now or is so urgent that you can't take the steps you need to be okay.

If you feel you're ready to do the work of addressing trauma, call forth a situation where you felt like the rabbit—where you lost your ability to fight or flee, and instead froze or appeased. Before you go any further, does this feel like something that you feel strong enough to work with on your own right now? If the answer is a yes, from inside your body, then go ahead gently. If you aren't sure, ask yourself if you would like to have someone, such as a trusted friend, guide you through it. If the answer is no, see if you could land on an experience that has a similar quality or dynamic to it, but that doesn't have as much fear or charge associated with it. If you feel that you need the help of a trained professional, reach out to someone in the resource section of this book. Then you can skip this next section, and we will join each other in chapter 7.

Allow your mind to travel back to that scene. As if observing from a bird's-eye view, imagine that the whole experience was laid out on a film strip. While you're scanning these frames, notice which ones you keep returning to—the ones that stick out the most. Notice the moments that feel like turning points, moments where there may be space for possible repairs. Now zoom in your awareness on the one frame that feels the most significant, perhaps the one that has the most charge. Be mindful to choose just one moment. Every experience has many moments, but we can do the best work when we home in on one moment. You can always come back and revisit this process with other moments.

Once you've landed on one moment, recall it in as much detail as you can. What was the environment like? What color were the walls? What did it smell like? What was the temperature like that day or night? What time of day was it? Who else was there? With your eyes open or closed, fill out the scene as best you can. As you fall into the scene, track any sensations or emotions in your body, and remember that you can go at your own pace.

Where were the other people in the room? You may feel a foggy and hazy feeling, as if you were starting to drift away. Notice that impulse, and return to the feeling of your legs and feet and the present moment. You may feel a lump rise into your throat, or your hands clenching, or a strange physical pain. Don't resist the urge to express these words or movements. Say the words out loud, or make the movements. Continue to sink deeper into it. Is there anything else about this scene that you could fill in, that you may not have noticed at first?

Softening deeper into this moment, maintaining your awareness within this specific frame, recall the physical position you were in at the time. You may want to get into that position now—whether you were lying on your back on a hospital bed, standing up over a sink, sitting in a restaurant chair, or walking as you turned your head to look behind you. Allow your physical body in this present moment to get into the shape it was in in the past in the frame you chose. Do so slowly, and notice what's happening as you transition into this new shape. Let your head and neck move around orienting yourself to the current moment space in this new position. Then, return to the scene in your mind, you in the scene. This alone may be enough input into your system for today. If so, stay with the sensations, emotions, other images, or movements that may be arising. Give yourself a lot of time and space. Let your body continue to regulate itself. Continue to breathe, tracking your current self with those past sensations.

If your system is feeling safe to take a next step, from this new physical position call to mind the person who was the perpetrator in this situation—whether friend, boyfriend, babysitter, family member, care provider, or stranger. Remember, we are still working within the one frame. Having them in the same room as you probably feels way too threatening, so put them as far away from you in your imagination as they need to be. In your imagination now, they can be on the other side of the city, they can be in another room with a cement or glass wall between you, or they can be in the corner of the room. Choose an option that feels manageable for your system. From this position where you are now, notice what's happening.

Are you in a freeze right now? Are you holding your breath? Do you feel cold? Are you drifting away? If so, don't force anything. Freeze takes time to thaw, no rushing. If the freeze is in your physical structure, as in you feel like a sculpture, allow yourself the space for breath and movement to start to animate your body again. Don't "make" yourself move. If you give your system enough time, it will show you what's next.

Remember that freeze was an adaptive state; to rewire it for the present moment takes presence. If you notice yourself dissociating, rather than fighting it, notice where you go, and how it feels where you are. There is probably something that feels good about where you go. This isn't always a literal place, although there might be one, like the ceiling or a corner or a certain distance from your body. It could just be a sense or feeling of "not here" or "no one home." You might feel light, or free, or safe where you go. As you notice what might feel good about leaving, let that sensation permeate your body. Land that blue. Let yourself integrate the positive sensations connected to it. Then you may start to come back and track the process of returning.

When you feel fully present in your body, within the frame, what is it that you are moved to do? Are there words that you want to say to this person, or just in general? It's really helpful when the words arise organically from the feeling-sense that you had in that moment, so hang out to see if the right words come to you. They don't have to be polite. These are the words your system wanted to say without protecting anyone else's feelings or experiences. So they don't even have to be anything you can actually imagine yourself saying in real life, but right now, in the scene you're in, let your body speak. There's a whole range of words that I've seen drop like a penny in the slot. If nothing arises organically, one of these might land for you. "I need more time." "Listen to me." "Stop." "Leave the room now." "I can do this on my own." "Don't look at me that way." "Back off." "Get away from me." "How dare you?" "Fuck off." When you say these words, you may notice that you have a reaction against saying them, or they barely squeak out. That's okay, just notice that. You also may have an emotional reaction. If tears come, let them come.

You also may notice that there is an impulse to move. If that impulse is clear to you, then go ahead and complete that action. If you are having a fight response, you might notice something small like a clenched fist or jaw, or you may have the desire to grab, punch, or kick. Allow yourself, both in your mind's eye and in physical reality, to slowly make that grabbing, punching, or kicking movement. Sometimes to feel satisfied and complete with a fight response, it's helpful to have something to contact. Something to squeeze like a pillow, something to push like a wall or a person. When I am doing this work in session, I give the person my hand or forearm to push or squeeze or kick. Having something to push against and activate that muscle pattern is what allows for the discharge and deactivation to happen. This takes a little creativity so that you can be in the position for the scene with the opportunities for contact with a prop or the wall. You might want to combine the movement with words. Integrate the fight response in movement, words, facial expression, and volume.

If you are having a flight response, like you need to leave, notice if it's clear in the scene where you would go. Would you get up off a table or bed? Would you go out a door, get out of a car, or go over a balcony? Sometimes the flight response and how you would leave may appear in the present moment—where you would leave in the space you are in. Either way, in your imagination, in dream time, allow yourself to complete that response. See yourself leaving. Watch yourself in your mind's eye making a successful escape. If it's not clear to you where you would go, slowly start to pedal your feet, as if you are walking. Moving your feet one at a time, see what happens in the rest of your system. Maybe there will be another emotion or impulse that follows.

There may be times in this process where you start to experience a sense of helplessness or resignation that may be reminiscent of the earlier experience. Allow for that, but also remember this is happening in your imagination right now. You do have the power now to make a different choice in your system that you didn't have then.

Check in with yourself. Has your system had enough? Making any of these shifts in your nervous system sets in motion a whole cascade of responses and changes throughout your system. Are you ready to change gears, to rest or go for a walk? If so, put this book down, and go do those things.

Words are written sequentially. I am limited while writing in terms of how I communicate this process to you, but you may have already layered this experience based on your own intuition and creativity. Just like the feeling of looking at a beautiful piece of artwork, putting on makeup, or knowing how to season your food, you have to trust your feeling-sense of when is enough. Err on the side of less, since most of us err on the side of more.

Otherwise, do one more scan. From the position where you are, in the scene that you're in, do you feel complete? Have you said what you needed to say and done what you needed to do? If yes, soak in that feeling of completion and satiation. If no, what else wants to happen? It might surprise you, it might be pulling someone close to you, or calling out for someone—there are infinite possibilities.

When you feel complete, even if it feels like there might be more for another time, slowly return to the here and now. Look around the space you're in. From whatever position you are in, take your time to upright yourself. At each stage of changing positions, orient yourself again. The process of coming back should take at least five minutes. This is integration time and it is critical for your system even if it feels unclear that anything is "happening." If, for example, you were lying down, roll to your side, breathe, and look around. Sitting up, breathe and look around. On all fours, breathe and look around. On your feet, breathe and look around. Allow your eyes to roam freely, as you notice both your inner world and your outer world, taking all the space and time you need to calibrate and integrate the experience you are having.

You may notice spontaneous words come to you, like "I can be here" or "I feel connected." Say them out loud if words bubble up within you. If no words come, try on the phrases "I matter" or "I can" or "I am powerful" to see if one fits, right now, in this moment. Only use these words if they feel true in your experience. These words are meant not so much as affirmations of a desired experience as they are a proclamation and declaration of your felt experience. This is the beginning of activating predator energy in your body.

Claiming predator energy can restore and embolden a sense of agency that is unwavering and incontrovertible. You matter, and you are powerful. Let the weight and strength of those words course through you, your muscles, your arms, legs, jaw, and back body. Remember your fangs. Inhabit your prowess. This agency is yours.

PART III

BODIES TOGETHER

THE SOCIAL NERVOUS SYSTEM LANDSCAPE

CHAPTER 7

MARKING YOUR TERRITORY

Defining Limits and Boundaries

A lioness separated from her pride and isolated in a cage will relentlessly trace the perimeter. She will fight against the bars, biting so hard she might break a canine tooth, injuring herself trying to get free. She may turn that restlessness inward and chew or harm herself. She may lie down and give up, as if sedated. Separate a mother from her cubs and she will experience an enormous amount of stress. Interrupt a mother animal birthing, nursing, or feeding, and that mother will do whatever possible to protect her young and her territory. When threatened, these animals will fight to be free of confinement and to protect their young, even at their own demise. Separation and isolation often feels like torture. And yet, for us human animals, our instinctual need to belong can keep us from fully being ourselves, or worse, keep us stuck in unhealthy or even abusive relationships.

The work we did in the last few chapters is focused on the process of reclaiming ourselves and beginning to nurture the full range of our nervous system's responses. We've addressed how to thaw out freeze responses, made space for flight patterns, and activated our fight responses. We've also learned skills to track those responses, allowing them to express themselves and move out of our systems. In order to activate these healthy sympathetic self-protective responses, we have to get underneath our social conditioning, beneath our inhibition and our morality. We have to dare to not be nice and polite, we have to dare to break unspoken rules, we have to dare to be bold about our needs and desires. We're ready to address our default social nervous system responses.

BELONGING, FAWNING, AND FITTING IN

When we feel safe in our social nervous system, we know that we can be ourselves, have needs, express our uniqueness, and still belong to our family or our community. We can be our wacky self and still be accepted and loved. A desire for proximity, an exchange of looks, touch, and play are all a part of being together with other mammals and feeling a sense of belonging. Remember that fight-or-flight responses happen in the sympathetic nervous system, and that the freeze response happens in the parasympathetic nervous system, in its dorsal branch, the back of the body. There are two more responses to threat that we need to add— *fawning* and *fitting in*. Both fawning and fitting in happen in the parasympathetic nervous system, in its ventral branch, the front of the body, which is also known as the social nervous system. We get into trouble when our belonging is or seems conditional on minimizing our unique expression, hiding our talents and gifts, or having to contain elements of our individuality so that we can remain in our family or social group. For many of us, we've mistaken or coupled belonging with fawning or fitting in.

Fawning is when we become nicer and less threatening in an attempt to de-escalate a threat. Just like we don't choose to fight, flee, or freeze with our rational mind, we don't choose this behavior consciously. It's crucial to remember that just like all nervous system responses, or default behaviors, fawning is an attempt at repair. In this position we are imagining the following: "If I return to this person who hurt me, maybe something different will happen and somehow erase what happened earlier. Maybe I'm confused and disoriented (freeze) about whatever transgression happened, and if I go back, I will somehow see that I was wrong and that painful thing was just in my imagination."

In its earliest stage, fawning manifests as niceness. The strategy goes: "If I'm really nice and polite, if I make myself cuter, maybe I won't get hurt." It progresses to appeasing and then acquiescing. The strategy continues: "If I lose my sense of personal wants and desires, I will be able to please someone else and I can stay safe." When your fawning response is activated, your body "believes" it's safer to stay close to a threat than it is to disagree, fight, or flee, even if your mind is in disagreement. Another less obvious fawning behavior is laughing as we speak to lessen the power of our words. We try to soften any potential conflict or rebuttal or retaliation by being nice while we're attempting to set a boundary. While we might judge these behaviors before, during, or after their display, they deserve some respect. There is a kind of intelligence at work here even if it is misguided by an unconscious social nervous system.

Fitting in is another response to threat. Think of how animals are camouflaged in their environment. Their skin and coats often blend in with their natural environment so that they aren't easily spotted by predators. Alternately, camouflaged predators are more easily able to stalk and attack prey. As humans, we have many ways to camouflage ourselves. We figure, mostly unconsciously, that if we stay invisible or small enough, we can avoid conflict. Think about it. We can wear clothing that helps us go unnoticed or blend in. We can talk quietly and only say things that are expected. We can hide behind technology instead of meeting with people in person. I hear many people say, "I need to put myself out there more," and then judge themselves for why they just aren't doing it. Remember, this is not a moral issue or a character flaw! Our defensive behavior of fitting in most likely was an effective strategy that kept us safe at some point—in our family unit, religious or spiritual group, workplace, or relationships—that became a habit.

Trying to fit in is a normal social nervous system response— but if that need is crippling you, if it's keeping you stuck in a bad relationship or a career that doesn't suit you, or causing you to hold your tongue when you want your voice to be heard, then it's time to recognize that fear is unconsciously running the show. As you bring these behaviors into conscious awareness, you can then slowly—as the nervous system always prefers— begin to make small changes to reveal yourself. And if fitting in is the *only* way that you can belong safely in your environment, then, surely it's time to explore new territory. Slowly, but surely.

We explore that new territory, and mobilize ourselves out of fawning or fitting in, by sensing our center, exploring our outer contours, and having a felt sense of our limits and boundaries. Developing the ability to hold your ground, increase your capacity to find your center among discord, and potentiate your capacity for conflict—while also maintaining connection—is where limits and boundaries become essential. The work on an individual level is to let go of the belief that having no boundaries will make us virtuous, mellow, spiritual, or easygoing. Our well-being actually depends on us setting defined limits and boundaries. There is a high cost to choosing the relative comfort and reward of fitting in over claiming your territory and belonging to yourself. In actuality, when you take a stand for yourself, the rewards are far greater—you'll start to find that you are in control of much more than you may have believed previously.

You might know in your mind what you deserve, like how you want to be treated in a relationship or how much your work is worth, but there's a gap between what you know you want and how you're actually going to get it. The way to fill that gap is to learn how to feel your own embodied boundaries, recognize a yes, a no, or a maybe *in your body*, and then practice the articulation of those impulses clearly. That's exactly what we're going to do now.

BOUNDARIES AND NERVOUS SYSTEM CAPACITY

When we remember to think of setting boundaries as a nervous system capacity issue, it can be a pretty straightforward practice. Our social environment has norms and its own capacity, so anything that makes us stand out, even if it's a good thing, can sometimes feel threatening. For instance, if you earn more money or you have more education than everyone in your family or community, that can actually register as a threat in your system. Your nervous system might unconsciously be "warning" you that you are too much of an outlier—that you aren't fitting in enough—and that might threaten your belonging. Likewise, if you earn less money than everyone in your family, that can also register as a threat in your system. Differentiating from the rules of your family, religion, or culture can register in your system as life-threatening, because fitting in to those groups' implicit codes of behavior has ensured our emotional and physical survival in the past.

Rationally, you probably know it's great to be yourself, break the mold, and live according to your own standards, but your body—your nervous system—may feel otherwise. Your body may feel a sense of fear, shame, and guilt about a desire you might have to *not* fit in, and in response, trigger some fawning behaviors.

The ability to speak and say, "I want," and "I need," is the one way to establish sovereignty. Sovereignty is like ruling your own one-person country—with limits and boundaries—and belonging to yourself, first and foremost. Your country has needs and desires, and resources to protect, and you are going to make them clear in your declaration of independence and interdependence! Rather than fawning, you can learn to become unapologetic about who you are and what you need. Rather than fitting in, you can learn to find your strong center and to stand your ground. In this way, you become like the queen of your territory and the protagonist of your own life, while also creating close and abiding relationships and allyships.

I've met very few women who find it easy to set boundaries without practice. Whether it's saying yes to one more thing when we're already overwhelmed, trading services or charging less than we can afford or deserve, or going along with someone else's plans or agenda before we realize it's not what we wanted for ourselves—we tend to allow others to set our boundaries for us.

When we're faced with questions about boundaries, we may default to the pattern of how asserting our individuality and desires worked out for us in the past. We've all experienced boundary ruptures, and there are typically two opposing strategies that we can adopt in response to those experiences. We tend to either open up the floodgates and let anyone in, or we batten down the hatches and rarely let anyone in. The response of opening up the gates is called "hypoboundaries"—your boundaries are loose and permeable. They might be nonexistent. Everybody can come in. You might think, "Nobody has ever listened to my limits anyway, so what's the point in even trying to have any?" Battening down the hatches and locking the doors is called "hyperboundaries"—your boundaries are so solid that they are actually impenetrable. Nobody can come in. You might think, "People always ignore my boundaries, so I am going to make them so thick that it will be impossible to reach me." Both of these defense mechanisms are understandable responses that occupy the extreme ends of the spectrum as our social nervous system tries its best to reestablish safety, relearn how to trust, and identify its own criteria for closeness.

You might already recognize how this behavior—setting too many or not enough boundaries—maps onto the sympathetic and parasympathetic tendencies. Someone who has a more parasympathetically driven system will tend toward hypoboundaries. Remember that people who are parasympathetically dominant tend to have more elastinous connective tissue. The tissue itself is less dense and can make it more difficult to perceive where boundaries lie, making us more likely to default to a "yes" response. Someone who has a more sympathetically driven system will tend toward hyperboundaries, being more challenged to let people get close to them. A hyperboundaried person has dense collagenous connective tissue and is more likely to default to a "no" response.

So how do we develop strong and yet flexible, fluid boundaries?

HOW TO OCCUPY YOUR OWN SKIN

On a physical level, the boundary between you and the world is your skin. One of my favorite facts about this organ (yes, skin is an organ!) is that the skin and the nervous system develop from the same layer in our embryonic development, the *ecto-derm*. Therefore, the skin is not only the most perceptible phys-ical boundary to define ourselves, it's also uniquely connected to our nervous system. Additionally, skin itself is not a uniform boundary, but a porous, permeable layer. How permeable your individual skin is is partly a function of the kind of connective tissue you have. Becoming aware of our own skin—through a felt sense—is an excellent way to learn to attend to your bound-aries.

Let's try a simple exercise right now. First, make sure that you have your feet on the ground. So either stand up or perch your-self forward on your chair so that you can feel your feet because I want you to be able to feel the ground. Go ahead and slide your feet back and forth on the floor. If you have a carpet, and you are sitting, then your feet might get a little hot from the friction. If you're standing, go ahead and shift your weight onto one foot and rub or scuff the opposite foot against the floor so that you're really feeling the sole of one foot, and then go to the other and do the same.

Now rub your hands together. Once you can feel the friction between your hands, bring them down to feel the soles of your feet. It might kind of tickle on your feet. Now put your hands anywhere you want on your body. You can put your hands on your face, on your eyes; put them wherever you want and just take a moment to feel the sensation: it might feel warm, cool, tickly.

So now we have the palms of your hands in contact with your skin. Take some time to slide your palms along your arms, your legs, your pelvis, your belly. Don't forget the back of your legs, your hindquarters, your wings. Feel the skin of your palms at the same time as you feel the skin on other parts of your body. See if you can become aware of this membrane, this organ—this literal boundary—that is separating your inner world from your outer world. Think of your skin as a magnificent boundary between you and the elements!

Then there is another moving "membrane" that is less visible, but possibly as perceptible as the membrane of your skin: you have an *energetic* membrane that can also be a powerfully effective and useful boundary.

Let's get a felt sense of this membrane as well. Place your hands in front of your shoulders and start to move your hands forward to feel the space in front of you. Where do you end and the world begins? Where is your space? Imagine defining your personal energetic space. It's not a literal thing, so there is no way to get this right or wrong. So if you were painting yourself inside the bubble of your space, let your arms move around in that space. Look behind you, too. And let yourself move and really paint yourself into your bubble of space. See if you can feel that. Explore pushing to the sides of your bubble. Possibly move your arms asymmetrically, beside you and behind you. You are defining an egg shape or bubble of energy that is around you, and discovering how close or how far away it is from your skin. Now explore slowing it down even more. Really focus on perceiving this membrane. For some of you, it might help to situate your eyes a little bit back into your head. See if you can say internally or out loud, "This is my space. I claim my space. I decide who comes in."

Now see if you can home in on a feeling of collecting and retrieving all the different parts of your body. Let yourself feel your body's spinal column, and then your sacrum. Go ahead and rock-pump your spine back and forth a little bit. Rock back toward your sitting bones and round a little, and then pump back. Now focus on feeling your feet connecting into that pelvic movement. So you're pumping your spine from your feet and you're letting your head follow. You can go as fast or as slow as you want. Let yourself experiment moving at different paces.

I want you to feel your feet almost like you're pushing and pulling them. If you're standing, you can do this bent over a little bit with your hands on your thighs so that you feel that you can pump more. Start with your pubic bone and your tailbone, and use them like a pendulum so that you're swinging and letting the rest of your spine go with you. You got this; there is no "right" way! Feel the power of your legs pumping. This is an exploratory experience, so you can explore however your body is asking you to move; but I want to really emphasize that you feel into your feet and into the space that's between your navel and your pubic bone. Have some fun bending your knees a little bit as you stick out your butt behind you.

If you're sitting, it's the same thing. I just want to suggest that you start to feel your quads fire a little bit. And when you bring your tailbone forward, bring your abdominals back. Don't think about when this process is going to end. Just let yourself live inside your spine and feel the rest of your body waking up—both front and back—as you light it up with your focus, breath, and imagination. Then if you want to move your arms, go for it! Opening and closing, opening and closing, and accentuating this movement.

Now it's time to come back toward stillness. You can make the movements smaller and smaller at first. If you're standing, consider sitting down, but you don't have to. Place your hands, both of them, on your lower belly. See if you can consolidate your energy into your body and inside your skin, which you are much more aware of now. If your thoughts are moving out in all directions like arrows moving centrifugally, then in your imagination, turn them back in and direct them all the way into the center of your brain, back toward your brainstem, all the way down your spine, all the way into a big and beautiful globe in your belly that is held gently in the bowl of your pelvis. Pull the energy in. See if you can imagine it and also feel it.

If you stop to feel your feet or your legs, slide your feet again. Shift your weight. I want you to feel the friction from the skin on the soles of your feet scuffing, like you're an animal that's rooting in the ground, or that wants to bury something. See if you can enjoy the feeling of pulling, and then feeling the rest of the back of your body light up from the movement.

At the same time as you're feeling this consolidation of energy, feel all these arrows coming back in. I am taking you through a deliberate and continual process of directing your mental energy back into sensing. Just keep redirecting your thoughts to sensations, movements, and feelings. See if you can imagine yourself diving beneath the thoughts as you move. There's really no limit to how far inside you can go, and how deeply rooted you can feel down into your heels, and down into your tailbone.

Now bounce a little bit. If you're standing, then you're just going to rock your feet forward and heel drop, heel drop, heel drop, heel drop, heel drop. If you're sitting, squeeze your glute muscles a little bit. As you squeeze, engage your legs, feel your feet as you bounce, bounce, bounce, bounce, bounce, bounce, bounce, bounce, bounce. Breathe. Inhale two, three, four, five, six. Exhale two, three, four, five, six. Inhale. Exhale. One more time. And then pause.

Notice any sensations.

Then come back to the layer of your skin. Use your hands to touch your sweet skin and remind yourself of that layer. Now notice what happens with your breath. Then extend your attention out around you remembering that bubble of invisible energy you sensed earlier by tracing it with your hands.

Now, some of you are probably thinking, "Well, my space is

different depending on where I am and who's around. If I'm on a train or an airplane, my space is different." That's true! There are material world considerations, of course. Maybe when your father-in-law comes around you'd rather that he stayed longer than at an arm's distance. Maybe you love it when your best friend comes up cheek to cheek. Your access to space and preference for space is definitely situational. What's not situational is that your skin will always remain exactly where it is as the membrane of your body. So consolidate all those molecules of your skin and pull those molecules of you closer so that your energy field becomes denser as well. See if you can go all the way to the ground until you feel your full coat.

A MOVING CENTER: DEVELOPING YOUR INTUITION

Knowing who you are, what you think, who you want around you, and how close you want them to be around you can be experienced as a fluid process: it shifts over time. Part of this fluidity is that there is no one boundary or rule that is going to fit for every situation. The good news is that you can practice and master this capacity to be flexible. You can practice finding your center, and returning to it again and again. In my classes, I guide women in different role-playing situations so that they notice how their body responds in real time to challenging questions and what their default reactions are. Then, when a similar situation arises in the future, they can recognize those earlier movements, sensations, or feelings, and they can begin to develop the capacity to communicate with their internal security system. By developing our felt sense of *knowing*—in our bodies—beneath what our mind thinks or wants, we mark our territory with a new consciousness that transforms our experience of living in our bodies.

Part of that new consciousness is learning to feel a clear "yes" or "no" in your body. What is your somatic boundary? How does "yes" *feel* in your body? How does "no" *feel* in your body? How often is the response fuzzy? I'm going to ask you to answer a few questions out loud. It may seem silly, but trust me, it's not. It's important because there's a difference between just thinking a yes or no and actually saying it. Speaking out loud becomes a declaration. Speaking out loud is also practice of moving from thought to action. A thought is an impulse inside of us; words are actions that move into the outer world. Speaking can be a bridge from insight to action, a mobilization.

Here is the first question: "Would it be okay if I came over and cleaned your house?"

Notice what happens in your body. And then respond verbally.

Maybe you feel a "hell yes." Maybe you feel anxious, or guilty, or burdened by the offer. Maybe you're thinking, "You're busy and you don't live close to here and I could never put you out like that." Or "I value my personal space and I like things a certain way and I don't want someone in my home touching my things." Where was there sensation in your body? What was the sensation? Is there an image you can use to describe the sensation? Is there a movement your body wanted to make?

Now go ahead and come back if you feel like you've moved away from your center at all. Just viscerally come back. Remember to turn the arrows back inward and consolidate your energy, by moving your attention inward and downward, especially to your pelvis, your belly, and your feet.

Here's another question for you: "I feel like I've got a lot of space right now, so I was wondering if I could give you a free session?"

How is that? What did it feel like to say yes or no? Do you notice any physical changes—did you start rocking back and forth?

Smiling? Did your lip twitch? Was there a sensation in your stomach? Did you get a little frozen? Did your biceps tense up?

Did you feel a clear "Yes!" or do you feel unsure of how to receive such an offer? Did tears well up in your eyes? Warmth in your heart? Did you wonder, "Am I allowed to just accept and receive that?" Is it hard to believe someone wanted to offer help? Does it make you feel excited? Or does it feel like you might owe something in return?

If you felt something like "Right now doesn't work for me, but some other time would be nice," do you actually want to do that sometime, or do you not want to, or you're not sure? Watch for those bait-and-switch responses—those ambivalent thought processes. For example, someone can set a boundary, but there's some other bargaining chip that they want to keep on the table. It's so important to know when we're sending mixed messages. For the purpose of this exercise, stay with the no. Feel where it lives in your body. This is so very crucial to be in touch with and know our "no"—to practice finding it and saying it. So often we might be afraid we're going to hurt someone's feelings or let someone down.

One more. Slide your feet one more time. Feel your spine a little bit. Open up your peripheral vision. Feel the back of your head. Feel the space beside you, behind you.

"Can I give you a breast massage?"

I'm betting that one caught you off guard.

Did it make you cringe? Cringing is really important because it's a retraction. Disgust is usually also a retraction. Did you feel a no? If so, where did you feel it? Did you feel uncomfortable, as if your space was being invaded? Did you feel you had to express interest in order to be polite?

There is no right answer to any of these questions. What happens, though, is that our neurons start to get all crossed up thinking that it's best to want it or not want it. It doesn't mean you're more progressive if your body did say yes, and it doesn't mean you're a prude if you said no. We're just simply listening for what our body says.

Feel where the yeses and the nos are in your body, and how they feel. Warm? Cold? Still? Moving? Pay attention to any qualifiers, too—ways you might be softening the yes or no. If you know where to look for a yes or no in your body, if there seems to be one particular area or signal that is speaking to you, you can check in there whenever situations arise that need your honed and embodied intuition. If the location or sensation of yes or no changes, that's normal, too.

One way of moving out of the fawning response is to learn to set limits and say no. When you feel that no, you'll begin to use phrases that begin with "I need" and "I want." You'll be able to identify needs that may be different from those of your boss, your parents, your friends, or your partner. When you notice that you're fawning, you can come back to your center, and check in with your true needs and desires. You can practice becoming decisive and clear with what your needs are and not afraid to differentiate. When you notice that you're having a fitting-in response, check in with that fear or shame, and choose to make baby steps in showing yourself; whether that means disagreeing with a family member, ordering what you want for dinner, or cutting your hair the way you like it, you can be confident in your self-expression, willing to risk a little to say yes to who you really are. You might be surprised that there are people in your life who will delight in the revelation of preferences and pronouncements that are more uniquely you.

Every animal knows how to find a water source and a food source—how to meet its essential needs. Embodied knowing is our own unique ability to meet our essential physical needs as well as needs for relational safety and connection. A deep and certain wisdom lives within you and it is best "heard" through your body. Uncovering this intelligence and developing the power to express your needs is an ongoing practice, but one that will give you the ability to know and articulate what is true for you at any given time and in any given situation.

CHAPTER 8

ATTACHMENT AND RELATIONSHIPS

How We Bond

Humans are social animals. We are dependent on one another for our sense of belonging and place in the world. We rely on each other as mirrors for our own experiences of life. In the last chapter, we began to strengthen our sense of sovereignty and center, minimizing our default social nervous system responses of fawning and fitting in. In this chapter, we will look more deeply into how we form bonds, and ultimately, create stability and a sense of belonging in a relationship.

In addition to the influence of our social nervous system wiring, we also bring our own unique attachment "style" to every relationship we have. If we peel back another layer of why it can be so challenging to set boundaries, we'll find that many of our habits in relationships are a product of our attachment wiring. Attachment theory, a theory of human bonding and connection first developed in the 1970s, offers us a fascinating framework from which to learn and understand our attachment style. I am not a psychologist nor an attachment specialist, but I do find attachment theory enormously helpful in understanding human relationship dynamics. I draw mostly from psychologist and marriage and family therapist Dr. Stan Tatkin's work, because he integrates principles of early mother-infant attachment with adult intimate relationships, as well as nervous system regulation—and that is the framework I will share with you here.

It was as a parent that I first became interested in learning about how attachment works. As I was parenting my daughter, I was experiencing a level of distress at times that seemed completely disproportionate to certain situations. I was also defaulting to what I thought was "attachment parenting," but instead was a kind of enmeshment with my daughter where I was unconsciously trying to repair my own early attachment needs. I realized that in some ways I needed her to need me. As I learned about attachment styles, I began to understand that my lack of awareness about my attachment style was influencing my daughter's development and the formation of her attachment style. With that understanding, I could heal attachment patterns in my own family line and start creating secure attachment for both of us. Then I found it so revelatory in understanding my own relationship behavior—not only in parenting but in dating, with my own parents, and in friendships—that I started covering attachment theory in all my courses.

The basis of attachment theory comes from the now-famous "strange situation" experiment devised by Mary Ainsworth, a pioneering developmental psychologist, in the 1950s—a procedure she conducted with thousands of mothers and babies primarily in Uganda and Baltimore to observe how babies and mothers reacted to being together and apart. The basic setup was a specific series of comings and goings, whereby a mother came into a room with her infant, then left the room, and a stranger came in, and then the mother returned. It was an 8 step process.

that a mother came into a room with her infant, and let her infant explore the space. Another adult, a stranger, then came in, talked to the parent, and then approached the baby. The parent would leave conspicuously while the stranger directed their attention to the baby. After some time, the parent returns, greets, and comforts the baby. Researchers noted things like how the baby reacted to their mother leaving and returning, how the baby reacted to the stranger, and if the baby continued to explore the space while their mother was gone. As well, they noted specificities of the mother's words, tone, and gestures, eventually correlating the two.

From these studies emerged an understanding of the three most common types of what are called attachment "styles"—*secure*, *avoidant*, and *anxious*. Stan Tatkin created three corresponding names for these types, which I love; he calls them anchors, islands, and waves. I'm offering an overview of these three attachment styles here because I think it is consummately useful to know where you fall on the spectrum of attachment styles as you're learning to work more consciously with your social nervous system. What is important (and exciting!) to bear in mind here is that these attachment styles are not foregone conclusions. While we do tend to fall into one category based on our relationship to our primary caregiver as an infant and child, our parents' attachment styles, and our early relationships, we can travel amid some of the behaviors of each attachment style over the course of our lives. There are also other categorizations and types that are more specific, like *anxious-avoidant*. I am choosing a simplified version because I have found that the majority of people do fit into these three categories. I want to help you better understand your attachment style(s), how your nervous system is involved, and how the resultant behaviors impact your boundaries in relationships.

When my daughter was a toddler, I didn't know anything about attachment theory or patterns. I had no idea that what I was feeling in the present moment could be connected to a sense of connection and safety I felt or didn't feel when I was her age—that my own attachment wounds would impact how I mothered her. Attachment wounds are the imprints we carry related to how we may have had difficulty bonding, the ways that our needs were not met in our relationship to our primary caregivers.

Healthy attachment isn't based on being perfect and never making mistakes or never being in conflict. In all relationships, including the parent-child relationship, we experience mis-attunement, conflict, and misunderstanding. The famous British psychiatrist Donald Winnicott documented such conflicts between parents and children, terming them *ruptures*. He suggested that parents can heal these ruptures through the process of returning to their bond with their child and repairing it—thus laying the groundwork for secure attachment with the parent as well as others in the future.

Attachment patterns are set in motion before we can even talk, and they live in our implicit memory. The way that our caregivers modeled the process of rupture and repair lives in our bodies. Attachment styles have a profound influence on the way we approach relationships throughout our lives, and by identifying and examining your attachment style you can gain new insight into your relationship dynamics. You can also repair attachment wounds in present time as an adult. Part of that repair is in the awareness of and respect for those early patterns that do get stirred up when we care deeply, as well as learning how to communicate those specific feelings and sensations, without trying to pretend otherwise.

This present-time repair work can be extremely effective in partnership and very close relationships. The prevailing model of relationship improvement used to focus on individuals working on themselves first, and then working on repairing their relationship together. Now that we understand more about attachment theory and also polyvagal theory, we know that some of the best repair actually happens *inside* the relationship. Our attachment styles and default patterns are activated within the context of a relationship, so many times the most effective place to heal them is in relationship. Attachment styles are not only relevant to familial relationships, romantic partners, and close friends—they can also impact our behavior in the most basic types of relationships, like those you have with the people you hire, your landlords, or your next-door neighbors.

For those who want to be in an intimate relationship or partnership and are not, understanding more about past and current attachment style can offer agency in this endeavor, as well as a key to understanding the behavior of prospective partners. Most of us have ideas of how we'd like to be in relationship—maybe we want to keep things casual because we want to protect ourselves from getting hurt, or maybe we expect that having the capacity to have sexual relationships outside of commitment or strong attachment should be doable, or maybe we'd like to be able to be more vulnerable and let someone in a bit more. It's important to recognize that any ideas of *how we would like to be with another* stem from a desire—a need—to stay connected to ourselves as we connect with someone else. Rather than trying to adopt the attitude of who we wish we were in relationship—a perspective looking from the outside in—attachment theory allows us to use an internal reference. By learning to be in an attuned relationship with ourselves first, we can learn to communicate to others from that internal knowing about what makes us feel safe and comforted.

DISCOVERING AND UNDERSTANDING
THE THREE ATTACHMENT STYLES

The first attachment style we'll explore is secure attachment. People who are securely attached are known as **anchors**. When an anchor's mother left the room, the baby may have been a bit distressed, but was able to calm itself down. The baby would acknowledge the stranger and then continue to explore the room. When the mom returned, the baby was visibly excited and would go toward her.

People who are securely attached often have relatively drama-free relationships. They have a lot of space for their partner to be who they are. They can be in relationships with the other two types, waves or islands, because they are steady. Anchors have a wide range of behaviors that they can tolerate without their own security feeling threatened. They feel securely attached within themselves, so the amount of distance or closeness their partner needs doesn't usually rattle them. Anchors don't get completely swept up in a relationship—the relationship takes up a healthy amount of space in their life, but it does not become their whole life. They have a wide capacity for solace and togetherness, finding ease in both independence and interdependence.

As parents, secure attachment is definitely what we're aiming for: to offer our children ourselves as a secure home base from which they develop internal security. However, life is life. Many factors can disrupt secure attachment and some of them are out of our control. Fortunately, like every other kind of trauma, there is always the possibility for repair.

The next attachment style is avoidant attachment—people who identify with this style are known as **islands**. As babies, islands didn't show any signs of distress when their mothers left the room. When their mothers returned, they either ignored them, or were ambivalent about whether to go toward them or wander off in the opposite direction.

Islands experienced an imprint at an early stage that their care providers couldn't be counted on to be there for them. Their care providers didn't respond when they did communicate their needs, so they stopped communicating them. Their care provider may have been depressed, been an addict, or had a lot of other children to take care of. Or the care provider could have been raised to value independence and therefore expected self-sufficiency earlier than was developmentally possible. In turn, the child developed habits of self-reliance. They learned that their needs wouldn't be responded to if expressed, so why bother? Island children can appear so effortlessly self-sufficient that even well-intentioned parents sometimes fall into the trap of reinforcing their avoidant behavior.

To those around them, islands truly seem like islands—like they could exist on their own and don't really need anyone else. Because they learned how to be detached from an early age as a survival strategy, as adults they fear engulfment and value autonomy. Their partners often feel like islands disappear or are not fully present; they may seem stingy with their energy and time, and retreat back into themselves for safety. Islands are the most capable of any of the attachment styles of having unattached or anonymous sex without it impacting them emotionally. They're afraid to expose their needs or desires too much, and avoid feeling dependent on others. Islands can be really picky—no one is good enough for them—which gives them an excuse to never get too close.

The final attachment style is ambivalent attachment, or **waves**. These infants showed distress before their mother even left the room—desperate and clinging. Then when the mother returned, they were either resentful or resigned and helpless.

Waves had caregivers who were sometimes highly emotionally attuned and sometimes completely unavailable. That unpredictability leads waves to feel anxious about whether a secure base is really there or not. They're not sure what kind of mirroring they'll get from their care provider; sometimes it's accurate and sometimes it's mis-attuned or nonexistent. Waves fear abandonment. They fall hard and fast, and they merge easily. They're often quick to trust, but then because they dive in so fast, they start to distrust. There is an internal feeling of pushing and pulling—quick to think that the other person is going to leave, or that maybe they want to leave. The doors and windows of the relationship never feel sealed tight. They want commitment but are always questioning if it's right and real.

Waves are the type most likely to engage in unsafe sex, because they want to feel a sense of depth and closeness more quickly. Craving closeness, they are more likely to use sex for relationship currency. They may go too far too fast, because they are unsure of how far they want to go and get in over their heads, only to feel exposed and vulnerable afterward. Boundaries are hazy for waves. Waves are likely to overgive, to stretch themselves for a relationship beyond where they feel comfortable—sometimes for the sake of a relationship more than for a relationship with that particular person. Waves can seem like they lack discernment because they're so eager to be in a relationship, and when they do find someone the relationship dynamic often takes over their life, making it hard to stay focused on other areas of their life. They are more prone to give up their routines and adjust their preferences to adapt to someone else's.

When my daughter was two years old, I would occasionally leave town for four to seven days to teach trainings or retreats. Having lived in three countries and eight homes in those two years—and being the only parent present in her life—she'd already developed a sense of insecure attachment. Our home and the circumstances inside our home were always changing. As much as I'd like to think of myself as a secure base for her, in those two years, I was recovering from a birth injury, struggling with breastfeeding, living in a new country away from my friends and family, separated from her father, and having to get real about making a living as a yoga teacher. All of these factors exaggerated my own waveness, my own ambivalent attachment. Of course, it has probably occurred to you that the very fact that I was even in that situation—a new relationship and a new country and a new baby in under a year—was due to my waveness! I jump in deep feet first and then sort it out later.

An island would dip one toe in at a time, while a secure person would feel no urgency or rush. For financial reasons and also to unconsciously repair my own attachment wounds—which I did not recognize at the time—my daughter and I shared a bed in our one-bedroom apartment. I felt that I was being an accurate mirror for her emotions, but in reality, I was hanging on to my relationship with her as everything else fell apart. She was my security almost as much as I was hers, but I didn't see that at the time. When I would call home from retreat while traveling, she would cry on the phone and become bereft. The people who were caring for her asked me not to call, said it was better for her. At the time it made sense, but now I know that it would have been better for me to call every day, even if she did get upset when I called. At two years old, she would then understand that I hadn't gone forever, and she would have the consistent check-in. It's been an ongoing process for me to help her become more securely attached, to help her self-regulate, and to also get the space that I need.

What was it like for you as I described the three attachment types? Notice how you feel in your system. Images and memories of certain people might be flashing through your mind, or you might feel a little uneasy in the recognition of your past behavior. See if you can stay with the sensations in your body without losing your center. If you are adopted, or experienced the death of a relative at an early age, or spent some time in the hospital as a child, try to allow this process to be encouraging rather than discouraging. In these cases, you are reviewing and remembering a potentially extreme attachment rupture. This knowledge may give you some context and insight into how these very early experiences impacted you, and what the imprints are in your nervous system. Now you can take that insight forward to consciously build the kind of relationships you want.

Just as people who are more parasympathetically dominant often partner with people who are more sympathetically dominant, people who are ambivalently attached (waves) often partner with people who are anxiously attached (islands). The relationship dynamics we choose are opportunities to loosen the imprints and cycle up into a new level of organization and repair, where we respect our past while creating a new present moment dynamic.

For example, my client Jocelyn is an island. She grew up in a family of mostly men, with a mother who struggled with mental health issues so was often unavailable. From an early age, she took care of her brother and cousins. She was a great student, got her first job at twelve, and rode her bike around town. She was praised for being so independent and competent. In her adult life, she is the breadwinner for her family and she travels all over the country for a job she loves, while her husband, Josh, works part-time and stays at home with their two children. She's organized and responsible, and doesn't understand why the satisfaction she feels with her own life seems like such a big problem for Josh. She thinks he has a pretty good life and wishes he would stop wanting more from her.

Josh is a wave. He was raised by a single mom. Sometimes he felt like he and his mom were a tight impenetrable unit; other times she was nowhere to be found, or unexpectedly combative. Her moods were unpredictable. Josh had never met a woman like Jocelyn, so self-assured and accomplished. Jocelyn loved how warm and caring Josh was and how close he was with his mom and family. Josh loved being with Jocelyn and wanted to spend more time together. That was a theme throughout their marriage. He wanted more intimacy and closeness, and she thought things were fine the way they were, if only he would be happier about them. Josh started to resent that she lived a whole separate life away from their family, and he was left to take care of everything at home. When he expressed that he wanted more closeness, it would happen for a short period of time, and then she would go back to her usual ways, of doing all the things that she loved to do, without considering him as much as he wanted to be considered. She felt put-upon by his requests. He felt shut out and taken for granted, not to mention slightly emasculated.

This is a common pattern with waves and islands. The bigger the wave gets, the more clingy, desperate, and desiring of connection and reassurance—the further away, the more unavailable and removed the island gets. Over time, Josh learned not to take Jocelyn's need for autonomy personally, and by doing so his waviness lessened. He learned to savor the time they did spend together, rather than losing himself in always wanting more. Ironically, his realization that "wanting more" came from an earlier pattern with his mom made him feel more secure in himself. And with that security, he stopped resenting Jocelyn and taking her behavior personally. He began developing more of his own interests and groups of friends; he learned to enjoy his own life separate from hers. Instead of resenting Jocelyn, he learned to feel more confident himself. Over time, Jocelyn learned that communicating more about where she was and what she was up to meant that her husband and children felt more oriented, grounded, and, yes, more secure! She discovered that it didn't lead to them encroaching on her time or taking away her freedom; in fact, everyone was happier.

CREATING SECURE ATTACHMENT

It's easy to idealize secure attachment and feel like we're messed up if we aren't "anchors." While it can seem like being securely attached is "right," and the other styles are "wrong," there are benefits to each attachment style. And besides, no human being is narrow enough to fit into one category and be defined exclusively by it. We are rich, complex creatures.

Waves are often artists, musicians, creatives, and healers. Waves are sensitive and can easily access spiritual dimensions. Islands teach us about self-possession and drive, unapologetically following the beat of their own drum and doing things their way. They are self-assured and don't require a lot of outside approval or reinforcement to stay their course. Islands are often planted squarely in the material world. So rather than feeling ashamed by or stuck in the type you most identify with, try to allow these categories to be informative and liberating. When you recognize your tendencies, you can make better choices, communicate your needs, and work on habits that aren't serving you.

Knowing your attachment style can be an important step in creating secure and trustworthy relationships. Understanding attachment styles may also help you understand the behaviors of those you're close to. When we are not well-differentiated—*when it's not clear what originates from us and what originates from the other person*—other people's attachment styles, and nervous system default patterns, affect us more strongly. We can have a lot more compassion for ourselves and the people we love when we recognize some of these patterns that might be unconsciously running the show. They're not choosing to be needy and clingy or distant and indifferent; their attachment tendencies are at the surface. When we notice ourselves being needy and clingy or distant and indifferent, that's a clue that we're not feeling safe. That lack of safety might not be coming from what's happening in the present moment. In fact, it's probably not. If it feels out of proportion to what's happening, like you're thinking that your boyfriend might break up with you because he hasn't responded to your text in the middle of the day, it's probably an echo of earlier attachment wounds. When this happens, orient yourself to your environment, allow for a deeper breath, and embrace the moment as an opportunity for repair of an earlier attachment wound.

Once you know your own attachment style—island, wave, or anchor—you can choose to communicate to others with that information in mind. Knowing yourself and telling another person about yourself, in this case, about your attachment style, can be very illuminating to both people. But you don't need to use the words "attachment" or "style." This can be a simple communication, like "Just so you know, I'm a person who needs a lot of space. In the past, I've been afraid of commitment, but I'm really working on letting down some of my walls. If you feel me pulling away, you can just gently tell me that's what you're noticing. I may still need some time on my own, but that doesn't mean I'm going away for good" (island); or "I want you to know that sometimes I need a lot of reassurance. It's vulnerable to say, but I get nervous when I don't hear back from you for a few hours after I text you" (wave). Being honest and letting someone know what is really happening for you can start to build trust.

In my experience, many women react to these suggestions by

saying that they have to trust someone first before they can reveal these things about themselves. While I certainly want you to let your intuition guide you here, I also suggest speaking up sooner, rather than later. We can create the foundation for the trust we want by having these conversations at the beginning of a relationship. If someone reacts harshly or discounts what you share, that's likely not a person you want to go deeper or share more of yourself with. That's useful information to have before you get too attached, possibly in an unhealthy way.

I've learned that creating healthy attachment has a lot to do with paying attention to comings and goings—to hellos and goodbyes. We can create and cultivate healthy, secure attachment in our relationships by paying closer attention to consciously marking and honoring our comings and goings. What better way to show our care and delight for each other than hellos and goodbyes? If you are sitting at a table working, when your child or partner comes in, look up and take the time to say hi and acknowledge them with eye contact and a smile. In the age of screens and headphones, this has become an even more important step, because it's so easy to not do it, and to get in the habit of not doing it. I think you will be surprised at how much things change when you really make a point of acknowledging these transitions. You also might want to include touch in these exchanges, offering a hug or a kiss with the greeting. We are relational beings and we need this kind of contact and reassurance—even the most securely attached among us! When you say goodbye, it's helpful to build a bridge to the next time you will see each other, even if it seems obvious.

For years, as a single mom, I struggled to pick up my daughter from school on time. Sometimes I would run late with a client and call my parents in a panic to see if one of them was closer than me to the school and could pick her up. Sometimes I would send a friend there when I was running late. My daughter was often caught off guard by who was picking her up. Later on, a wonderful au pair came to live with us. For the first couple of months, I would pick up my daughter whenever I could. I knew drop-offs and pickups were important, and I wanted to do them. But I fell short with all the other projects and clients I was managing. So I decided that it would be better for our au pair to do all pickups, so that my daughter would know what to expect. I still sent her off to school in the morning and kissed her goodbye as she left the house, and I would find her wherever she was in the house with a big smile and hug when I got home. She told me that she felt much more relaxed and secure knowing what the plan was every day and that the plan usually didn't change. This was a conscious attempt to repair a rupture and recreate a secure attachment by bringing in another trusted caregiver to provide a steady and reliable presence, even if it wasn't me, her primary care provider. It takes an attachment village to raise a child.

"Good mornings" and "good nights" serve not only as important bookends to the day, but also as a way to create continuity of connection that is foundational for strengthening bonds. While these may seem like little things, they go a long way toward making everyone feel safe, calm, and cared for. Marking comings and goings, orienting to the structure of the day and to each other, creates predictability and stability for our social nervous system, knowing that we belong, that we have our people. We regulate ourselves and co-regulate each other with these ritual greetings.

You might remember from earlier chapters that the social nervous system evolved from maternal bonding. The attachment repair that we've discussed here is essential social nervous system strengthening, and also a way of creating a stronger, deeper safety net of support. These little rituals help us to trust ourselves and trust others; they create the sense of belonging that binds a community. We don't have to go back to our family of origin to heal attachment wounds, although the conscious implementation of these rituals would no doubt be impactful there as well. You don't have to rehash your childhood or rely on the participation of your parents to heal attachment wounds. You can start from wherever you are, with your relationships and interactions in the present moment. You can do it with coworkers. You can do it with your best friend. You can do it with your child.

Establishing habits and noticing your own behaviors in communication and closeness is the path to creating more securely attached relationships, which is ultimately settling for your nervous system, as you widen your net of social support, where you can truly express your needs and desires and be heard, as well as be able to hear the spoken and unspoken needs of others. Then you are out of the realm of gameplaying, interpretation, and cat and mouse. You are in the realm of genuine human connection without posturing and pretending.

A hallmark of secure attachment is regular and consistent communication. Reliability creates a secure bond, an understanding that settles the nervous system. Depending on the relationship, that might look like anything from a weekly check-in to chatting on the phone several times a day—whatever is decided upon, you can set clear expectations about communication. Does that sound unromantic or lacking in spontaneity? Perhaps. But once you experience the deep satisfaction and comfort of a secure attachment, you'll realize that there are a lot of other ways to create spontaneity than to keep your system on edge all the time, wondering if a relationship is reliable.

THE LEVEL OF RELATIONSHIP

Our addiction to intense feelings and experiences often surfaces in our relationships as well. Last year, I went on a date with a man, and we hit it off. We agreed to see each other the following week, which I was excited about. The next day, my date sent me his work schedule. He continued to message me, and then got frustrated when I didn't respond. I could see that he was distressed, and since I am committed to this attachment work in all my interactions, I try not to react or distance myself based on another's distress. So I let him know that I had been working when I got his text and I didn't feel that I needed to know his work schedule. He said he was sharing his work schedule so that we could plan out all the times that we could spend together going forward. This felt like too much—a wife needs to know your schedule, not someone you went on one date with. I told him I'd see him the following week like we'd planned, responding but also holding my own boundary of the amount of communication that felt good to me based on the level of our connection. He grew so frustrated that he told me he didn't want to see me again. It was clear to me that he was experiencing a rush from our initial connection and wanted to dive all the way in from day one—a classic wave behavior. Being a wave myself, I have learned to titrate my way into relationships. I am still enthusiastic, I enjoy the positive parts of being able to connect easily and deeply, but now I lean back a little more. I have learned that slowing down helps me to be able to hold on to myself and see the truth of what and where a relationship is rather than where I want it to be.

The reality is that while it can feel great to fall for someone quickly, healthy relationships take time to develop. We need to experience things together to build trust and connection. Our bodies need to get used to each other to build intimacy. This doesn't mean that you might not have a "feeling" about someone. It just means that the more we allow a relationship to ripen at a digestible rhythm, where we hold on to our own path at the same time as we get to know someone, the less likely it is to backfire or implode dramatically. In general, the nervous system appreciates pacing. It likes to take a few steps and then rest and look around, and then take a few more steps and notice the view, and then maybe do a sprint and take a nap. When we respect the pace of our nervous system, we do less backpedaling, we have fewer blowups, and we avoid unnecessary conflict. When we respect the wisdom of the nervous system, we also don't end up somewhere we may not want to be without knowing how we got there.

If you've dated for any length of time, you've probably encountered someone who seems to enjoy having the power to keep you guessing, or being unavailable—or maybe you've been that person to someone else. Yes, there's a temporary reward for remaining aloof, trying to act like you don't care, but you can't have a great relationship presenting something you're not from the beginning. Pretending can only last for so long. And the power you get from pretending isn't the truly satisfying power that comes from a deep, connected bond.

When we feel unsafe because of a new situation, however good or bad, when our nervous system is challenged by that novelty because we have stronger feelings than normal, the shadow side of our attachment style is likely to flare up. We may feel so good, and care so much, in a way that we're not used to, that we text someone fifteen times in a row to clarify something we said on the date, or conversely, we might never contact them again. As we move toward secure attachment, be aware that it takes some time for default patterns to change. When we're used to the adrenaline and drama of pushing and pulling, hard-to-get, cat-and-mouse games, secure attachment can seem boring or flat in comparison! We literally have to train our sweet nervous systems to not only trust, but also enjoy predictability and accountability. If "connection" in our family of origin was unpredictable (wave or island), then understandably, reliable connection will feel unfamiliar at first. It will take time.

There's a difference between meaningless small talk and scouring, soul-excavating exchange. If we don't share ourselves at all, there's no juice, but if we share too much, we can experience a shame hangover. You might notice how this relates to boundaries. Islands tend to be hyperboundaried, and waves tend to have fewer boundaries, and therefore are more prone to oversharing and then feeling regretful later. It's helpful for waves to practice containment, and perhaps not share as much as they might normally. They can learn to hold their cards a little closer to the chest. It might feel uncomfortable, because they're used to the catharsis that can accompany sharing. But a wave can remember that they're lovable and worthy of relationship just as they are—they don't need to prove their worthiness. And it's helpful for an island to practice softening their boundaries, to allow themselves to express their emotions and to share what they care about. An island can remember that just because they express affection now doesn't mean that they're signing on a dotted line for commitment!

All of the labels and terms in this book—from parasympathetic to sympathetic, elastin to collagen, downregulation to upregulation, hypoboundaried to hyperboundaried, waves to islands—can be used as tools for self-understanding through inhabiting our nervous systems more consciously and completely. We all fall somewhere on a spectrum of these opposites—nothing is fixed.

An attachment style is not a life sentence; it was an adaptive strategy that you unconsciously developed as a child. Knowing your attachment style as an adult can help begin the process of repair. It can help you stop idealizing how you "should be" in relationship, and instead, become aware of the potential pitfalls of your attachment style, so that you can develop an ability to self-regulate when you are able, or reach out for the support you need from others for co-regulation. You can create secure attachment starting right now, right where you are.

CHAPTER 9

MORE FREEDOM IN SEX

In a move that proved to be very strange timing, my daughter and I relocated to Brooklyn in 2019, the year prior to the COVID-19 crisis. The move from suburban San Diego to the big city appealed to both of us. We wanted to be around more people doing things their own way—and what better way to experience extraordinary self-expression and cultural saturation than living in New York. But by mid-March of 2020, we were sheltering in place and school went online. There were no subway rides, no serendipitous interactions. The ease of public space in New York City became strange and contentious as we navigated what was safe with changing rules and information at the local, national, and global level. There were sirens all day and all night long, and we began to know people who were sick or dying. Friends began to close their businesses.

In late April, when we were being inundated with warnings about the dangers of contact with other people and most kids in New York had not seen their friends in several weeks, my daughter, then twelve, logged in to school one morning and found she was going to have sex education. I was dumbfounded. Under normal circumstances, we already teach sex separate from care, touch, relationship, intimacy, and communication—not to mention pleasure. We teach the reproductive mechanics and genital anatomy in two dimensions devoid of coming-of-age complexities, real-life considerations, and felt sense experiences. On top of all this, to have sex education during a time of great duress, stuck at home alone, our collective nervous systems in a heightened state of danger and fear, and unable to go within six feet of another human being, epitomized to me how out of touch we are as a culture with our sexuality. Is it any wonder that we find ourselves in a cultural moment where sexual boundaries and consent are confused, contested, and hyperintellectualized?

Contrary to what my daughter, and most of us, learned in school, I believe that sex is at the center of our human experience, so much more than a reproductive function you can learn about online. We can resolve a lot by looking there. Most of us have thought of sex as separate from the rest of our lives, separate from our minds, separate from spirituality, separate from our relationship dynamics. Many people don't talk about sex with their therapists. Many people don't talk about sex even with the people they're having it with. I believe we could learn a lot by turning this paradigm inside out and imagining sex to be the most foundational, and elemental, territory of our lived experience. We could learn a lot by treating our sexuality with reverence and respect.

All of the material we've explored so far—inside-outside awareness, pendulation, TIMES, attachment styles—can not only help you become more contented and at home in your own skin and develop more secure attachment with others, it can also help you expand your possibilities for sexual pleasure and erotic fulfillment. This work has helped to tone your nervous system so that you can support more charge and experience novelty with curiosity rather than alarm. It can give you the ability to track your sensations and to communicate what you want and need. As you expand your capacity, that communication will increase coherence in your facial expressions, words, head carriage, and spinal position. You will be able to orient in and out of your personal experience, and back and forth with another person's experience.

I've noticed in my work, as well as in my life, that in this time of redefining what we want out of sex and relationships, there's a lot of confusion. Many women are disoriented because while marriage is still somewhat of a social standard, there are so many ways we can be in relationship; we don't have a singular model for how things should go. We're carving out new norms, building the ship as we sail it, literally figuring it out as we go along. We've identified a lot of what we don't want, but we aren't sure how to feel for and express what we do want, especially in real time.

The work of this book aims to help you narrow in on those wants, desires, and expectations. We all get to decide how we want our sexuality to look and feel. We get to decide who we're going to share it with. We get to decide how few or how many partners we have. We get to determine if we want sex to be at the center of our lives. We get to change our minds. We get to grow and shift our preferences. While all of these are choices, trauma can limit our choices. Rationally speaking, you probably know that these decisions are yours to make. If you've experienced sexual trauma, you might be thinking, "Yes, theoretically those are options for most people, but not for me." I understand, and I assure you that it is possible to access these options fully if that's something you want to do. I know because I have helped thousands of women along their path to this freedom and because I have experienced this type of resolution in my own life as well. There are so many reasons and circumstances in which our nervous systems limit our options to choosing fully expressed sexuality. For example, some women I've worked with have experienced a dramatic change in their sexuality after childbirth, others have been limited by their experience of ongoing abuse by family members, and still others were confused about why they can't find a partner and an orgasm at the same time.

Great sex requires us to occupy the full spectrum of our nervous system range, from predator to prey—from healthy aggression to healthy surrender. If we are habitually the "rabbit," we're never the subject of our experience. We might slide into toleration, acquiescence, or collapse—default behavior—instead of easing into true surrender. If we have the capacity to occupy the predator side of our nervous system (healthy fight), we can be an active participant in the shape of our experiences, and decide if we want to be submissive. Just a reminder that the capacity to occupy the predator is different from actually acting as a predator and it is also different from desiring that role or wanting to be in charge. A felt sense knowing that we *could* activate our inner predator if we needed to, not just in sex but in our lives, is what gives us the larger sense of safety to then be able to truly relax or surrender. We can lift up out of our social nervous system training, and dare not to fit in or to fawn. We can repair our tendencies toward avoidance (flight) or helplessness (freeze) by developing the healthy fight side of our nervous system.

With access to the fight side of our sympathetic system, we can truly allow for surrender, the healthy expression of the parasympathetic side of the dorsal system. When we do this, we have more choices available to us of how we want to engage. Arousal energy is activation energy, so we can expand our ability to feel safe, stay present, and trust our own evolving boundaries as well as our capacity to communicate them by increasing the amount of erotic charge we can hold and enjoy in our system. Then, contrary to what we might think, we don't get stuck in one role all the time. We also don't end up in the same dynamic, same routine, and same predictable destination.

Sex is a topic that's been shrouded in secrecy and shame for many of us. Most of our sex education has been paltry and piecemeal. This chapter could be an entire book, and I will recommend many great resources for you to continue to explore.

UNRAVELING THE TANGLED KNOT OF SEX

The most important thing to know as you build your capacity to hold erotic charge and have better sex is to understand how we humans *couple*—that is, unconsciously link all kinds of things with sex and our sexuality. When my daughter was almost three years old, I realized—finally and for good—that a relationship between me and her father was not going to work out. My mind would have continued on, because it made more rational sense to stay together, to keep our family unit intact, and to keep trying to make it work. In my body, there was no other option but to leave the relationship. It was in leaving this relationship with my husband that I realized how much had been unconsciously coupled with my own attachment style, relationships, and sexuality. I had to begin to dismantle my deep wish and fantasy of the family I wanted and always thought I would have: one where there was one mother, one father, and children, until death do they part. I also had to begin to unravel all of what was caught up in my identity as a divorced person, and what it would mean for my daughter to have parents who weren't together. I became increasingly aware that my then-husband would likely distance himself not just from me, but also from our daughter. I saw that he wouldn't be able to separate his role as a husband and lover from his role as a father. He had unconsciously coupled romantic relationship with fatherhood. Clearly, I was having to make this painful decision for both me and my daughter.

I was going to have to unwind what relationship meant to me, and define my own values about how to form connections while raising a growing daughter. I realized I would also need to confront both my own inner stereotypes and societal standards of what it means to be a good mom, a single mom, and, yes, a sexual mom. While these may be slightly different questions than the ones you posed in your life right now, I'm sure that you've had your own reckonings about what a relationship means to you, and where and how sexuality fits into your life. Each of us has our own erotic identity, that when made conscious can actually be part of our deeper healing work.

Each of us also has the unique task of unraveling—and maybe also uncoupling in places—the tangled web of sex that includes the strands of attachment, pleasure, touch, feminine energy, masculine energy, play, companionship, and desire. When we're unaware of what's driving us, we may enter into each potential connection with so much unconscious charge—emotional and erotic—that things derail quickly. Things might go sideways because we end up having sex when we're actually looking to fill other unmet needs; those needs unconsciously may be overshadowing the reality in front of us. For example, we might end up going way beyond our threshold or capacity for sustainable connection, as we pendulate out of loneliness or disconnection and go into what we presume is connection, diving in too far or too fast. Or we may avoid or be threatened by true intimacy, having coupled emotional unavailability with love in our earlier lives. If we can identify each of these facets of our sexuality, and even untangle some of them, we might actually have the chance for new kinds of relationships. Conscious relationships. We can actually discover what's driving us so that we can be more straightforward and clear in our communications—honest with ourselves and, therefore, honest with the people we meet.

THE ROAD TO BETTER SEX: BUILDING YOUR CAPACITY TO HOLD EROTIC CHARGE

Our ability to stretch our capacity for holding charge is central to our ability to generate arousal energy, experience orgasm, and feel and hold pleasure, sexual or otherwise. If you've ever had sex with a man who can't hold an erection for more than a few minutes before ejaculating, what you're experiencing is a nervous system that can't tolerate—hold for long—a sympathetic charge. Or maybe you've felt like you would like to be able to have a more full-body, expansive orgasm, but it's hard for you to hold too much sensation. This is a woman's version of not being able to tolerate—hold for long—a sympathetic erotic charge. The answer here is to learn to not push ourselves longer, faster, and harder (sympathetic). Instead, we can practice pendulating between the sympathetic and parasympathetic sides of our nervous system. We don't need to insist on more activation and upregulation to experience deeper and more enduring sexual pleasure. Instead, we need to stretch the pendulum swing in the direction of downregulation, in order to get a fuller range of sensation, pleasure, and erotic possibilities. Pendulating grows our ability and capacity to create erotic charge, relax into it, and then distribute it, and to repeat that cycle.

When thinking about our capacity to hold charge, it helps to organize our hormones into two categories: sex hormones and stress hormones. The human body can't produce sex hormones and stress hormones at the same time; the body prioritizes which hormones to produce based on the messages from our nervous system, and they are reciprocally connected. If we're producing stress hormones, we'll produce fewer sex hormones. If we produce more sex hormones, we'll produce fewer stress hormones. If you're stuck in the stress modes of your system—in fight, flight, or freeze due to incomplete cycles from your past—you will produce less of the feel-good hormones.

The good news is that when you consciously turn your lens toward pleasure, toward anything that feels good (not just sexual pleasure), you can start to light up your sex hormone circuitry. So by deliberately doing things that feel pleasurable, and cycling through the channels of TIMES to imbibe all the ways they feel good and savoring those experiences, we begin to create more pleasure hormones. More pleasure hormones means fewer stress hormones. Pleasure is a powerful antidote to stress.

We can be better aware of how sex is lighting up our hormonal systems by knowing about these two categories—warm sex and hot sex. Warm sex is connected, golden, juicy, sensuous, and rolling, and it could go on forever and ever. Hot sex on the other hand is experienced as electric, fiery, full of suspense, and all about chemistry. Hot sex is adrenaline-based. Unfortunately, most of what we've been taught or seen portrayed about good sex is hot sex alone. We can learn to enjoy and experience the full range of both warm and hot sex.

From the nervous system perspective, arousal builds through cycles of upregulation and downregulation—a combination of sympathetic and parasympathetic engagement. Climax and ejaculation are sympathetic responses, but as we learned from the principles of pendulation and the expansion of capacity, trying harder and doing more don't help us to let go into the experience of our sexual pleasure—and the elongation of that pleasure. More pushing, grinding, focusing, and contracting is not what expands our capacity for sexual pleasure. So for many people who don't experience orgasms, it's not about having more focus and determination to access their desired pleasure and release, it's about expanding their capacity to downregulate, to relax, and to distribute sensation throughout their bodies, as charge builds.

Holding more charge than we are used to can feel scary and like we are losing control. Part of the reason that orgasm can be elusive is that it requires that we both build trust *and* lose control—that might include making noises, facial expressions, and movements, as well as saying things that do not come from your rational mind. That's part of why I led you through the practice of losing inhibition in chapter 6. Learning to let our bodies take the lead and trusting that, and getting used to our own sounds, helps us to move outside of our normal range of experience. While rationally we might be wanting something very much—whether that's to orgasm, or to feel connected while we orgasm, or to have spiritual sex, or to have multiple orgasms—we have to first learn to help our body develop a sense of safety and then slowly we can begin to stretch into new edges of erotic pleasure and charge. Don't worry—feeling uncertain can be a part of the process of you building capacity, always in a titrated fashion.

At this point, I want you to also remember the principle and practice of zooming in and zooming out. Moving from focused awareness to open attention is very important for expanding and extending orgasm. If you zone in on the genitals, and especially the clitoris, and imitate a male arousal trajectory, making more contact, harder, for an extended period of time, you aren't giving your female system a chance to expand and develop the ability to hold charge. By understanding the way in which the female nervous system is wired somewhat differently, you learn to slow down some so that you can feel arousal climb and then pause. You breathe, allow the arousal to spread throughout your body, and relax into it. Then you return to the experience of the climbing arousal. This is called *edging*—you are edging closer to climax, again and again, without going over the edge into orgasm just yet. Edging helps you extend your orgasmic range. While you are edging, experiment with movement. During the pauses, you can actually get up and dance or shake or make noises or change your breathing rhythm! Let your wildness emerge.

See if you can release the place that you think you want to get to, the fixation on the destination or goal, and let yourself be present to the pleasure along the way. It's totally possible to build your platform of arousal, so that you may climax in a way that doesn't deplete all of your energy, making you feel totally done, and sometimes hypersensitive to touch. When you build this kind of platform, you're building your tolerance for sympathetic charge with stimulation, as well as stretching your healthy parasympathetic range in the pauses. You expand the range of your pendulation, and by doing so, your window of presence widens. You can extend that presence and capacity for pleasure so that the climaxes don't drain all the energy from your system. Instead of a kind of sexual burnout, you can continue through your day filled with orgasmic energy.

THE SEX EDUCATION WE NEVER GOT

There are a few basic pieces of biology I want to explain before we go any further. Most of the information we received in sex education classes is predicated on a male arousal trajectory. And it is still standard fare for our kids. Male arousal is obvious because it's visible—a penis, external to the body, becomes hard and changes shape. Typical male arousal can take thirty seconds to one minute. Did you know that female bodies have just as much erectile tissue as male bodies do? Here's what was left out: genital arousal occurs—in male and female bodies—when the erectile tissue in the genitals fills with blood, swells, and becomes engorged. In female bodies the tissue is distributed differently. The erectile tissue in the female body lives in the robust clitoris whose legs extend internally along the labia, the perineum, the G crest, and the sponge that surrounds the urethra, and is mostly internal. The appearance of a fully erect vulva is visible and noticeable, if you look. All of that tissue can engorge, and full typical female arousal takes between thirty-five and forty-five minutes. Ejaculation for female bodies is just as possible as it is for male bodies, although it's been outside of our education, because female ejaculation isn't obviously relevant to reproduction (and as such, is still contested!).

Sex education tends to be specifically focused on reproduction, so pleasure mechanisms aren't addressed or considered relevant. Many women have never had penetrative sex that lasts thirty-five to forty-five minutes, which means many women have never experienced penetration with full arousal. Having penetrative sex without full arousal can be uncomfortable and even painful, and doesn't allow women to experience the full spectrum of pleasure and orgasmic experience that many are longing for.

Our sex education also ends up being slanted toward the male experience and the heterosexual experience, since the male contribution to reproduction is visible and more obvious, and because there is bias in how the science of reproduction has been written. In the same vein, the ideas that many of us have about how sex should go are based on male arousal style, as well as a heteronormative definition of sex, which is referred to as "PIV"—penis-in-vagina sex. All sexual acts are built around this main event of penetration, which makes everything that is not PIV an accessory to the main event, which is considered "real sex." The word "foreplay" itself suggests it is a precursor to something else, rather than an event unto itself. Foreplay is just something that has to happen on the road to "real" sex. This automatically places male pleasure at the center of the experience. Similarly, the words "climax" and "orgasm" have been used interchangeably. Climax is the dive off the cliff, while orgasm is the steady undulating climb of underlying energy that can be held without being discharged. Is it any wonder that women feel limited in their sexual experience with such a rote and partial road map? We need better language to express the complex totality of pleasure and sexuality.

Pornography, which is mostly made by men, for male consumption—with few notable exceptions—presents another challenge to the true breadth of sexual expression and possibility. The pornographic script follows the same trajectory, where you see the arousal building, picking up speed, harder and faster and harder and faster until the climax, and the sharp drop. Even women who are masturbating in porn are often imitating that same pattern, going increasingly harder and faster with an exclusively genital focus. There is almost no pausing, changing direction, allowing for sensation to be distributed, zooming out to contact the whole body, and the slow wave-y build typical of pleasure and activation in a female arousal trajectory. Pornography also rarely shows people who love each other or even pretend to love each other while having sex. What is depicted in porn is power plays and performances of fantasy, based largely on the male erotic makeup.

Lately the stakes have gotten a lot higher with pornography, which hits the rewards center of the brain. Some men who watch pornography regularly experience erectile dysfunction in real sexual encounters because they've uncoupled connection with arousal. This means that their stress hormone circuitry is primed while watching pornography. In order to have an erection while in a true human experience, they need to escalate the sense of danger, the forbidden, and the taboo. The content of what people are watching doesn't necessarily reflect their actual desires or fantasies; it reflects the escalating amount of charge they need in order to get the same dopamine hit.

Porn has also established some norms for the appearance of female genitals—creating yet another unreasonable and homogenized expectation. A woman's vulva is usually presented as a hairless outer labia that enfolds the inner labia and clitoris. In reality, vulvas are as varied as faces. The vulva, also known as the "vagina's neighborhood," describes the entire female genital area; vulvas differ in hair color, skin color, labial size, clitoral visibility, proportions, and size. All vulvas are capable of an immense amount of pleasure that has nothing to do with how they look—and yet, these standards create anxiety for many women. I hope we can all start to focus more on how our vulvas *feel* than how they look. Focusing on how we look keeps us in the default programming of our social nervous system, while focusing on how we feel can take us deeper into the experience of living in our bodies, with a greater possibility of increasing our pleasure—sexual or otherwise.

In my practice, I see firsthand the negative emotional effects of our culture's obsession with PIV. So many women feel guilty about needing or wanting foreplay. They tell me that they feel bad about taking so long to get warmed up, and taking "too long" to have an orgasm. Many women also tell me that they lie there and wait for it to be "finished." When I ask, "Finished with what?" they tell me they're waiting for the man to ejaculate. So, what I often hear is that foreplay is something they feel pressured, either internally or externally, to get out of the way in order to get to the main event, the main event being men's or-gasm. No wonder so many women are frustrated. Other women come to me with low libido, not understanding why they're not that interested in sex. Most of the time it's not that they don't want sex, it's that *they don't want the sex they're being offered*, and they don't know where to start with creating an experience that goes any differently than the usual script.

We've been told that we're wired for survival and that com-petition is the main driver of our nervous system, but thanks to polyvagal theory we know that collaboration and connec-tion, too, are essential for our survival. If we know that humans are indeed wired for connection, then we have a big project and edict in reframing the teaching and experience of sex as pleasure-based, something that has moved beyond reproduction as its purpose. It's an evolutionary shift—we can go beyond pro-creation into connection and pleasure, which we now know is also inherent to our survival and well-being.

THE AROUSAL SCALE: HAVE A SOMATIC CONVERSATION

Another way that I have found to create coherence as well as truly fulfilling connection is to develop the ability to have a so-matic conversation. Sharing in the present moment what you're noticing can undercut a lot of the stories we tell ourselves and assumptions we have. Many women share with me that they don't like how their partner approaches them. When their part-ner comes up behind them and hugs them while they're doing dishes, or gives them "the look" across the room, they immedi-ately want to avoid contact.

One strategy I offer women who find themselves in this situ-ation is that they use a scale of 1 to 10 to rate their arousal—1 being "I am not aroused at all/am almost asleep/don't want to be

touched right now" and 10 being "I'm excited and ready to go"—
and use this to communicate with their partners. After sharing where you are, and hearing where your partner is, you can
decide if you want to try to meet somewhere. In other words,
you may be at a 2, and they may be at an 8, but you're interested in moving in their direction, if they can meet you slowly
and stay in touch about where you are. Or you may be at a 2,
and your partner's at an 8, and you really want them to dial it
down to your range so that you can cuddle on the couch and see
where things go. Generally speaking, making overtures toward
sex requires some vulnerability, and most of us don't like to be
rejected. This also applies to setting limits and making requests
once we're engaged in sex—the fear of rejection can inhibit us.
Afraid to expand our capacity, we stay in a safe zone of our habits, and that rarely leads to exploratory, expansive sex. We get
into patterns of assumptions that keep us from having genuine
interactions in the moment, where new things could happen.

So using TIMES, here is how you might work with your partner
the next time they give you that "look." Notice your reaction—
the "look" (movement) that they are giving you has a meaning
(thought) for you. To you, that movement may be coupled with
a kind of sex you are tired or bored of. Your partner does not
know that unless you tell them. "You know, when you give me
that look, I automatically go into high alert, because to me it
means you want to have sex right now. And the sex it usually
leads to is totally different than what I want now." Then your
partner can orient to where you are and what's happening for
you, instead of making their own meaning, such as she never
wants to have sex and she's not into me anymore.

You take the lead to tell your partner what it is that you *are*
open to. If it's true, start with "I want to be connected to you"
or "I want to explore intimacy with you." Find a statement in

the social nervous system that assures your partner that you do want to be next to them or in communication with them. Then orient your partner by sharing how you're feeling. "I'm frustrated because I know what I don't want, but I'm not sure what I do want." Or "I'm afraid to tell you how I feel because I know you'll be annoyed or feel rejected." If you don't know how you're feeling, or you often state your feelings, then describe a movement or a sensation. "I notice that every time you give me that look, I look away from you, and my stomach gets tight." It's important that you're honest about how you're feeling, what you are sensing, or what movements you're noticing *in that moment*, not a report of past feelings.

Then get curious and listen to what your partner has to say. What are they open to? When they gave you that look, what did it mean to them? If being together doesn't lead to PIV sex, will they be satisfied and do they still want to participate? You might both check in on the arousal scale. Then together discover the parameters of how you want to be together. Is there a time constraint? Is there something that you definitely don't want or do want? What are the instruments that you're bringing to this improvisation? What are you totally game for? Now that you know where your arousal level is, what the parameters are, and what you're both up for, take action.

Here are the steps: slow down, connect, orient (you orient them), listen (they orient you), find a common point of interest and curiosity, define your parameters, share your limits/ boundaries in common, make an action.

This might seem like a lot of work. It might seem unfair that you have to lead the interaction. My experience is that this is a part of healing. We rise up into healthy sympathetic action. We have agency, instead of feeling put upon and slightly collapsed or defeated about having to say what we want and how we want it (parasympathetic helplessness). We can actually spiral up into a level of maturity and sovereignty where we enjoy communicating about what we like and how we like it. It takes practice, and we will make mistakes. Remember, there will be ruptures, and there will be repairs—that's a part of relating. This also might seem pretty cognitive and verbal for a book that's about getting beneath the level of thoughts to unleash organic impulsive desire. When you learn to have a somatic conversation, you might find yourself talking less in circles that feel like they go nowhere and habitual conversations without new openings, and instead learning new things about yourself and your partner. You might find yourself having present moment conversations that feel evolutionary, that lead to positive reparative experiences—not just smoothing over those record skips, but creating whole new songs.

MANY DOORWAYS IN

The best sex is like a jazz improvisation session. You bring your instruments, your desires, your quirks, I bring mine, and then we see where it goes. Sometimes we play a song or two and that's enough. Sometimes it's really flowing. We're experimenting and new sounds and songs emerge that we hadn't ever thought about. You don't make great music all the time, and sometimes it blows your mind. Great sex is a practice, like learning a language or an instrument.

And yet many of us feel we can't orgasm unless we're playing the same song in the same way over and over again. I've spoken with women who have said they can only orgasm in a certain position, or if they have one particular fantasy in their minds. If we take the same road every time, we get stuck. If your climax requires certain repetitive qualities to be enjoyable, each

experience will feel the same. The qualities that make for a fulfilling erotic life are curiosity, creativity, and novelty. We can
find new pathways and new doorways of discovery and genuine
interest. A healthy nervous system is one that can change direction.

Remember the description of trauma as being "too much, too
fast, too soon"? In creating reparative positive experiences,
which all of us need, we can do less, slow down, and take our
time. When creating new pathways and the possibility for new
riffs, pausing is one of our most important tools. In chapter 7,
we worked on limits and boundaries and what "yes" and "no"
feel like in our body. Pausing is what allows us to tune in to our
genuine impulses, to decipher what our mind wants, what our
body wants, and what is in alignment with both.

Many of us have felt that if we enter into a sexual encounter,
we have to continue until the end—the end usually defined by
male ejaculation. Because of the usual steep climb of the male
arousal trajectory we've seen and are used to, a desire to change
directions or pause is usually interpreted as a stop. I invite you
to bring the language and knowingness of pauses into your sexual connections. Pausing and stopping are two different things.
It's important to gain clarity in whether you want to stop or
you want to pause. You may need to pause first so that you can
know what you want. It's as simple as saying, "Can we pause
for a moment? I need to catch up with myself and take in everything that's happening." What you feel in the pause can inform
if you want to stop or if you want to continue. Of course, stopping is totally okay, too. It's important to listen to the difference
between tolerance and enjoyment, and stop when you are tolerating. It's important to know when you are satiated, so that
you don't override that signal and keep generating more charge
than your system can handle. When you've taken in as much as

you can digest and assimilate for that period of time, you can communicate that you "feel complete" or that you're ready to transition to another kind of relating.

I've noticed that after I introduce pausing into interactions, my partner learns by example and often asks for the pauses. It's easy for all of us to operate on autopilot, or get caught up in a fantasy, a performance, or a habit of how we've always done sex. Pausing allows us to get current with ourselves, with each other, and with each moment.

In order to do that, we need to throw out as many of the images and ideas of other people's versions of what looks good or hot or sexy and find our own definitions. We have to move beyond the fitting in and fawning defaults of the social nervous system to connect with our own individual sexual nature and slowly release our fears of rejection, looking stupid, or being weird, so that we can play and have fun.

We can also use the tools of TIMES to move ourselves to another spoke on the wheel. If you're always in the image channel with the same fantasy, what would it feel like to switch to movement? If you're never in the image channel, what would it be like to invite an image into your experience? Many people feel disconnected during sex and don't know how to come back into connection with their partner. Sometimes that's because we're stuck in one channel while our partner is in another one. For example, if we're in emotion, feeling tender and open-hearted, and our partner is deep in sensation, we might invent a meaning that they don't care, are selfish, or are in their own world. Instead of assuming, we can ask them what channel they're in. We can notice how deep in the channel they are or we are, and then decide to join each other in one or another channel. They can come to us in affect or we can move into sensation. Or we can decide to stay in our own channels.

We come into connection through communication, and rather than guessing where our partner's attention is and what we're imagining to be true about their experience, we can just get actual information. It can also be fun to start a sexual experience with the exploration of one channel as the compass. For instance, you could choose sensation, and be exquisitely attuned to the physical sensations of your skin and contact. Or you could choose image and the sound channel. You could experiment with different kinds of music, not just your typical slow jams—although that's fun, too—to see what that evokes in you. TIMES is an amazing framework to expand your creativity and doorways into expansive unexpected experiences.

BEING FULLY ALIVE

Most women have a sense that sex could be so much more than what they can access or experience. This curiosity and knowingness often lies hidden, disguised in half-expressed sentiments, without a place to live, without words to express it, and without a way to channel that knowing. A lot of the women I work with hope that a partner might be able to lead them into new territory, or they long for a place they were able to reach with a past partner.

Good sex begins with owning your body, becoming intimate with your external and internal landscape. From that place of self-knowledge and with the tools in this book, you can have good, if not great, sex all the time. That's possible because you know yourself and you know how to communicate. Slowing down allows you to take a TIMES journey with your own pleasure. If you caress yourself, feel your own breath, whisper to yourself, move slowly, you will get to know your own arousal. Arousal may stir emotion, all kinds. Arousal may rouse images.

Arousal can take unexpected paths and move you from the inside out. Arousal can bring incomplete loops to the surface, giving us an opportunity to complete them. For many women, reclaiming the predator is an experience of firing up their arousal.

Your sexuality is the foundation of who you are—the low hum undercurrent of being alive. Learning how to track the thread of pleasure—to ride the waves—and then riding those waves all the way down the backside is the key to owning and taking pleasure in your sexual experience. And why would you want that, other than because you're supposed to want it? Because orgasm, when we grow the capacity for it, not only is a source of pleasure but can also serve as an organic nervous system cleanser. Much like the "vu" exercise we practiced in chapter 5, orgasmic charge travels through the circuitry and shakes things free, makes things known that were unknown, and expands our sense of what's possible.

There's no magic button I can tell you to push that will improve your sex life, just like there's no one exercise that can heal your trauma. There are many resources out there that provide guidance on the mechanics—tips, tricks, and techniques—a top-down approach to mastering sex. What I offer you here is something that simultaneously taps you into your own resources and widens your capacity for experience—tools that you can use for the whole of your life. This approach is focused on sensing your system and what it truly wants, needs, and craves from moment to moment. This is the inside-out, bottom-up approach to an expansive relationship with sex. What's most important is the process of coming back into your body, which we've been working on all along. We've been knocking on all these doors hoping that one of them will crack open and one of them will make sense. There is an unlimited world of pleasure and connection awaiting. Will you answer the call?

FROM PERSONAL TO COLLECTIVE HEALING

The teachings and practices in this book are about learning to be fully human—dropping beneath the surface to the magnificent intelligence of the body and what it needs to do to unwind itself. The body is always there waiting for you to listen, to discover its wisdom, and to lead you to a greater sense of organization and congruence within yourself, with others, and with your environment.

Part of becoming human in these times is a process of getting to know your nervous system, coming home to your body, learning how to filter experience, expanding your capacity for pleasure and learning to reside there, and coming into wholeness with boundaries, communication, and sex. You have everything you need right now to call all the parts of yourself home and into greater coherence. Every life experience, every imprint, has brought you to this point to offer you the information you need to become the truest expression of your soul's purpose.

What is the call of the wild? It is unconditioned expression. It is innate power. It is the awakening of instincts. The call of the wild is an invitation to freedom—to hear who you are and be who you are, not who you think your mother, father, partner, or child wants you to be, or who you think you should be. The call of the wild implores the untamed and undomesticated you.

When you heed the call of the wild, you have more power than you think you do.

Awakening your own power allows for the possibility that you can develop the capacity and stamina to use that power and privilege for the collective good, not just your own. You spend less time on your own pain and trauma and have more available energy to look outside yourself. Your personal healing can fuel the collective healing. The outcome is more play, joy, laughter, pleasure, and receptivity, as well as the ability to shoulder more sadness, grief, and heartbreak without going down with those big emotions. We can occupy the range of feelings as we disrupt and reorganize the social structures that don't allow the full range of human expression, including play or pleasure, for everyone. When we feel safe enough deep down, when our capacity is so wide, we can weather the storms of conflict and the messiness of the redistribution of power without defaulting to our habitual trauma responses.

We have reached a moment of urgency that calls into question the power dynamics of healing itself—who has access to healing and how healing really works. One-on-one consultation with a healthcare provider, while highly desirable and even necessary in many cases, is an inadequate solution for the level of personal, cultural, and planetary imbalance at this time and simply not accessible to everyone who needs it. The skills and technology of orientation, directing awareness, landing in what is working, activating our predator responses, acknowledging our attachment strategies, and coming into wholeness need to become available and widespread to everyone who wants them.

Having been on the journey of this book, you are now equipped with jaguar skills, with a deeper felt sense of understanding of your nervous system and the nervous systems of others. As such, you can be a messenger of this new language. You can become a part of the redistribution of resources and of what has been considered specialized knowledge. You can help usher in a new era, where cancel culture and punitive redress are not the go-to tools. You can become an advocate for the voice of the body—yours and others'. You can become a living example of what it feels like to be around someone who has the capacity to locate themselves and return to their center amid a conflict or storm. You can become a stalwart accomplice. You have the tools to be a force for good, because you have a trustworthy center. So continue to do this work to make your center palpably robust. We need your compassion, discernment, and ferocity to move through and beyond assumptions, blanket generalizations, and compulsory beliefs, beyond the simplistic categories of "good" and "bad," "us" and "them," "victim" and "perpetrator," to create a world that respects the needs and safety of all nervous systems and all bodies.

At the time of this writing, we are five months into a global pandemic. There are many external safety measures in place as protective strategies for collective health, like sheltering in place, wearing masks, and social distancing. People are having a range of responses, from denial (freeze), to blaming others or the government (fight), to moving away from particularly affected areas (flight). There have been many incomplete cycles—deaths not able to be mourned, births and graduations not attended, family reunions canceled. Attachment challenges are flared, as people default to their self-protective patterns—like being overly clingy or disappearing. In trauma language, this pandemic would be considered an inescapable attack. It's unique, though, because in other inescapable attacks, the threat is visible—a dog about to bite you, a car about to hit you. In this case, the virus is invisible. We cannot see it. As a result, we are doing a tremendous amount of work as we move back and forth between the immediate physical reality, where things around us may look mostly normal, and the neocortical reality of remembering that there is a pandemic, so it is safer to be physically separate and there are things that we want to do that we cannot do. Each day, we have many impulses we can't follow to completion and satiation, because our brain reminds us that it's not safe.

My plea is that we do not become habituated to these safety measures. They are highly functional during this time, under extreme circumstances, but not functional at all as ongoing protocols for relating. By the time you are reading this, there will have been some big shifts in our physical mobility locally and globally. I cannot finish this book without enlisting you in one more way to be an ambassador for the organic intelligence of the body, and as such, a harbinger of a new era. As humans, we are adaptable and resilient creatures. And we are also able to adapt to things that are familiar or functional short-term, even if not in our best interest over time. We are able to become habituated to our imprints.

During this pandemic, many of us took our work, family gatherings, celebrations, and even dating online. Even if uncomfortable, we learned to relate with masks on, from a distance, and in many cases through barriers. While that has been necessary for this time, it is not at all optimal, for who we are as human animals, as a primary way of relating. External safety measures can never be a substitute for a felt sense of internal safety. After a long period of isolation and varying degrees of immobility, we are going to have to titrate our way back into contact. Just as adopting masks and limiting contact was hard for most of us to adapt to, so will be returning to relating in person, out from behind the masks.

We are not designed to thrive in isolation. We need touch. We need closeness. We need contact. We need to gather. Not only in the aftermath of the pandemic but also moving forward as a society, we need to feel we belong to ourselves and to each other. We must build the world we want to belong to. The way forward is—as always—together. Have courage!

ACKNOWLEDGMENTS

This book simply would not exist without Dr. Peter Levine's original insights on animal behavior, trauma, and the nervous system as well as his dedication to practicing and teaching the Somatic Experiencing work worldwide, and specifically in Brazil, where I embarked on this path.

Nan Kenney—you gave me my first taste of this work, and from that moment, I knew I was in an entirely different universe from the one I had known, exponentially potent. You also exemplified loving boundaries in a way my system had never felt.

Ale Duarte—you encouraged me through example, through inclusion, through transmission, through radical adherence to felt sense, and through countless "hold-it moments," which is your term.

Dudu Esteves, you gave me Jaguar—you stalked me, challenged me, witnessed me, and gave me this key. Neither of us could have understood the starburst of energy in that transmission, not just for me, but for the thousands of women since, and into this work. *Muito, mais muito obrigada.*

To all of the SE assistants and community, thank you for the wide net of felt sense support. To Lama Tsultrim Allione and Pam England—mothers and spiritual teachers, your work made this work possible.

In reverence to the indigenous and earth-based cultures who had (and have) original technologies before there was a need for codification. Thank you to Resmaa Menakem for building a bridge between personal and collective healing, bringing race to the forefront of somatic conversation, and forging connections in his book *My Grandmother's Hands* that I had not yet made but was desperately craving. I am here for the long game of the nine generations of work.

The writing of this book required a wide and emergent social nervous system in order to come to its full fruition. Stephanie Tade, wise advocate agent, imbibed the idea right away, and maybe more important, understood me. She also knew that Colleen Martell would be the right collaborator. Colleen—when I asked if I should interview more people, thank you for blushing and saying "no," claiming your place in our work together. We went through a full life cycle—fertility, pregnancy, birth, and postpartum of an actual baby in the middle of a pandemic, all while fiercely coming back to the center of what this book wanted to be. Thanks for wrangling the Jaguar when necessary! Harper-Wave—my dream publishing house—I knew from the minute I stepped in there it would be the home for *Call of the Wild*. Julie Will—thank you for your wisdom and generosity, and for not getting totally weirded out by a mini Rolfing session at our first meeting! A giant thank-you to the whole Harper team—Karen Rinaldi, Brian Perrin, Yelena Nesbit, Emma Kupor, Sophie Lauriello, Leah Carlson-Stanisic, and Robin Bilardello—for bringing

Jaguar to life in its truest form. There is nothing like the thrill of a collaborative vision. Reis Paluso brought enormous relief by translating my sketches into beautiful and clear graphics. Thank you for your support, patience, meticulousness. Thank you to Katrina McHugh for workshopping so many of the ideas and original sketches, as well as being an OJ—original Jaguar.

Jessica Murphy, my trusted assistant, kept the business wheels turning, making it look easy—the steady drumbeat through the twists and turns of the process and life in the time of cholera.

Some of my oldest friends circled to support me in various phases and stages to give me perspective, and turns out they are some damn good editors. Katie Friedman, historian and sex therapist, generously reviewed the first draft, giving me attuned feedback and revolutionizing the way I viewed edits. She highlighted the parts she loved, which allowed me not to fall in the pit of all the corrections. I returned to those words and sections often to keep me on track. I look forward to returning the favor! Chrisandra Fox, beloved yogini mama co-conspirator, shined her light, clarifying especially chapter nine.

To my Ice Tribe—Reis, Daniella, Cole, Roeshan, Lindsay, Justin, Brian, Mike, Luke, Marisa, Adrienne, Judy, Jeff—who gave me the first real felt sense of sangha—the real belonging, where you can be as freaky as you wanna be and still belong, with zero preciousness. To the men, thank you for holding down the masculine for me when I needed it most. To Daniella, for the bathing suits, pajamas, and constant thoughtfulness and encouragement.

To Kasper van der Meulen, for facilitating epic, soulful gatherings and trainings and for teaching from your heart. With great pleasure, I will rock a white board with you any day. Anna—for depth, hugs, soup, and being one of the first readers.

To Frank—for embodying the most crystal-clear fight response I have ever seen that has become a reference point, and aspiration.

To Dyana Valentine, for holding the seen and the unseen.

To Shannon—for the walks, guidance, understanding, love, and astro-magnificence. You have always seen the vision.

To Monisha—for the love and the fire, for the imagery and the trust.

To Juna—for steadily guiding me with love, for seeing the soul of the book, and of Jaguar, again and again.

To Tobin—my beloved soul ally, king of the image channel, devotee of connection, you teach me through your being and I am so thrilled that we now meet on even ground.

To Alicia—for being my Monday morning steady, and for steadily confusing me, keeping me a curious student.

To Raquel—thank you for walking the hard path with me.

To Deb—for teaching me about the possibility of friendship and healthy attachment.

To Circe and Charlie—for all the love, laughs, outrageousness, mutual admiration, and giving my crew a family home.

To Jennifer, Jeff, and Mollie—for welcoming me into your home when I came to do session work in New York, and welcomed us again when we moved. For caring about the evolution of session work, celebrating each stage of this project, and laughing a lot along the way.

To Alysse and Dan—for bedrock believing, deep belly laughs, and ever-evolving dreams.

To Sue—for taking care of me in the small ways—the fancy drinks, delicious meals, looking straight through me, and keeping track.

To Cristal—for teaching me from the beginning and becoming a dear confidante.

To Keli—for being tethered to the "blue," to always seeing the bigger brighter future, and stretching me with you.

To Tema—for your ferocious embodiment, transparency, devotion, and storytelling.

To Kris—for your tender and powerful heart, I am in awe.

To Agatha—for seeing and believing from the beginning.

To Nick—for being a clear mirror with the biggest heart and trusting me with your family.

To Miranda—for bringing the art, the understanding, and the flow, and chronicling the Jaguar mothering journey.

To Jorge—for all of our projects and explorations together, and for understanding what beauty really is.

To Ana Maria—we are undoubted kindred spirits. I knew that from the first time I saw your paintings. It is a dream come true to have your work on the cover. Thank you for being a quarantine auntie to Cece and sharing your gifts with her, too.

To Val—you weren't just Cece's *au pair*, you were also mine. For two years you cared for both of us, you woke up with a joyous spirit, and you reminded me that everything has its own time. You made this possible and sometimes enjoyable.

To Rahi—for walking your path so gracefully and being a steady presence in mine.

To Tanisha and Nia—I am so thrilled that we have adopted each other.

To Liz—for showing up, caring about the integrity of my soul, playing with me, pushing me further, and representing the opposite to make the center ever more clear.

To Sabia—for your confidence, brazenness, and brilliance. Thank you for making the work your own, living life on your own terms, and continuing to grow as a leader. Your voice is so needed.

To Matthew—ours was one of the most fortuitous meetings.

The value of you answering your phone sometimes every single day is immeasurable. I needed your voice, your listening ear, your wise counsel, your honest revisions, your knowingness, and your wonderings throughout this past year. I am so grateful.

To Carly, Prairie, Pam, Kiana, Shannon, Caitlin, Jamie—for courageously walking this path and restitching the fabric of this lost art of womancare, together. This is your legacy too.

There are a few people who were there from the very beginning to the end of this process. Ash Robinson, you have seen the whole climb. You are my steady cheerleader, my strategist, you held me through the first book's process and here we are seven years later—mothering and creating. I will always be your #1 hype woman. Sil Reynolds, brilliant crone, queen of hearts, sat with me on Zoom, and said over and over, "I have time for this," "I'm right here," melting shame and doing attachment repair in real time as we combed through revisions together. Your way is woven through the chapter heads, your presence felt throughout. Maggie Rintala, you are my ride-or-die, up-for-anything, acronym-brainstorming best friend. You met me on Zoom and in-person for daily workouts when that's what I said I needed the most. You know this material from the deepest inside, watched me as I developed it and women digested it and applied it, and shepherded the process of the courses and the book. You met me in all of my questions, and your voice is very much a part of this book. You made things seems possible, when I wasn't sure they were.

To all the women who've been in the Dome or on the table and to all the Jaguars—you are bold, brave, and inspiring. You are leading the charge in parenting, relationships, financial sovereignty, evolutionary sexuality—to redefine and resituate language and culture. We are here for the long game, the changes of equity, justice, and resource allocation for many generations. We are healing backward to heal forward. Your trust, courage, and ferocity move me each and every time.

To Mom and Dad—you have loved me through my worst, when I felt sure I was unlovable, and at my best—a real unconditional love.

And finally, to Cece, thank you for loaning me to this book. May it pave a path for the world that you want to belong to. Some day you might believe that this was for you. You are forever my heart.

FEELINGS LANGUAGE (FROM NONVIOLENT COMMUNICATION)

Feelings when your needs are satisfied is another way of saying "blue" feelings.

Feelings when your needs are not satisfied is another way of saying "red" feelings.

FEELINGS WHEN YOUR NEEDS ARE SATISFIED

AFFECTIONATE
compassionate
friendly
loving
openhearted
sympathetic
tender
warm

CONFIDENT
empowered
open
proud
safe
secure

ENGAGED
absorbed
alert
curious
enchanted
engrossed
entranced
fascinated
interested
intrigued
involved
spellbound
stimulated

EXCITED
amazed
animated
ardent
aroused
astonished
dazzled
eager
energetic
enthusiastic
giddy
invigorated
lively
passionate
surprised
vibrant

EXHILARATED
blissful
ecstatic
elated
enthralled
exuberant
radiant
rapturous
thrilled

GRATEFUL
appreciative
moved
thankful
touched

HOPEFUL
encouraged
expectant
optimistic

INSPIRED
amazed
awed
wonder

JOYFUL
amused
delighted
glad
happy
jubilant
pleased
tickled

PEACEFUL
calm
centered
clearheaded
comfortable
content
equanimous
fulfilled
mellow
quiet
relaxed
relieved
satisfied
serene
still
tranquil
trusting

REFRESHED
enlivened
rejuvenated
renewed
rested
restored
revived

FEELINGS WHEN YOUR NEEDS ARE NOT SATISFIED

AFRAID
apprehensive
dread
foreboding
frightened
mistrustful
panicked
petrified
scared
suspicious
terrified
wary
worried

ANGRY
enraged
furious
incensed
indignant
irate
livid
outraged
resentful

ANNOYED
aggravated
disgruntled
dismayed
displeased
exasperated
frustrated
impatient
irked
irritated

AVERSION
animosity
appalled
contempt
disgusted
dislike
hate
horrified
hostile
repulsed

CONFUSED
ambivalent
baffled
bewildered
dazed
hesitant
lost
mystified
perplexed
puzzled
torn

DISCONNECTED
alienated
aloof
apathetic
bored
cold
detached
distant
distracted
indifferent
numb
removed
uninterested
withdrawn

DISQUIET
agitated
alarmed
discombobulated
disconcerted
disturbed
perturbed
rattled
restless
shocked
startled
surprised
troubled
turbulent
turmoil
uncomfortable
uneasy
unnerved
unsettled
upset

EMBARRASSED
ashamed
chagrined
flustered
guilty
mortified
self-conscious

FATIGUE
beat
burnt out
depleted
exhausted
lethargic
listless
sleepy
tired
weary
worn out

PAIN
agony
anguished
bereaved
devastated
grief
heartbroken
hurt
lonely
miserable
regretful
remorseful

SAD
dejected
depressed
despair
despondent
disappointed
discouraged
disheartened
forlorn
gloomy
heavyhearted
hopeless
melancholy
unhappy
wretched

TENSE
anxious
cranky
distraught
distressed
edgy
fidgety
frazzled
irritable
jittery
nervous
overwhelmed
restless
stressed out

VULNERABLE
fragile
guarded
helpless
insecure
leery
reserved
sensitive
shaky

YEARNING
envious
jealous
longing
nostalgic
pining
wistful

SENSATION LANGUAGE

This list is the beginning of building your sensation vocabulary so that you can have somatic conversations. Add on to the list if different or new words come to you!

Airy

Bloated Blocked Breathless Brittle Bubbly Buzzy

Calm Clammy Cold Congested Constricted Contracted Cool Coursing

Damp Dark Deflated Dense Disconnected Disperse Dizzy Dry Dull

Effervescent Electric Empty Energized Expanded Expansive

Faint Flaccid Floating Flowing Fluid Flushed Fluttery Fragile Frantic Frozen Full Fuzzy

Heated Heavy Hollow Hot

Icy Inflated Itchy

Jagged Jittery Jumpy

Knotted

Light Limp Liquid Luminous

Moist

Nervous Numb

Open Overflowing

Paralyzed Pounding Pressure Prickly Puffy Pulsing

Queasy Quivery

Radiating Ragged Raw Restricted

Shaky Sharp Smooth Spacey Spacious Spinning Still
    Streaming Stringy Strong Suffocating Sweaty

Tense Thick Thin Throbbing Tight Tingly Trembly
    Tremulous Twitchy

Vibrating

Warm Wiry Wobbly Wooden

JAGUAR GPS: A GUIDED PRACTICE MAP

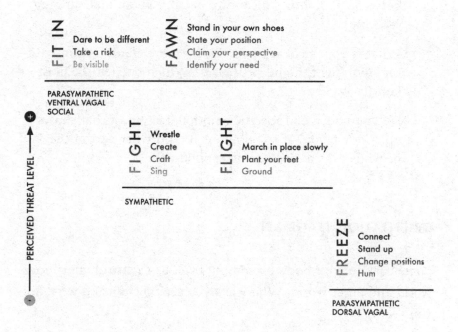

After you've read this book through, you may find that you want to return to the somatic practices.

The explorations in this book are sequenced so that you slowly build nervous system capacity. Now that you have explored them in sequence, feel free to experiment in a way that feels right for your body. Using the practice map here as an easy reference, you can go back to the practices that your body craves, or the ones your mind knows you need.

INNER WILDERNESS FIELD GUIDE (PAGE 3)

To set the foundation for healing work, it is helpful to identify your resources, both internal and external, and to notice your nervous system habits.

- Make a list of the things that light you up, that you love, and that make you feel good—the simpler the better (e.g., lighting a candle, petting an animal, singing, walking).

- What is your primary nervous system default response (fit in, fawn, fight, flight, or freeze)? Which one felt the most familiar to you?

- Do you notice one specific emotional signpost that shows up a lot for you? If so, which is it, and what part of the nervous system does it correspond to?

ORIENTATION (PAGE 35)

Come back to your body by coming back to a sense of your inner world and outer world. Where are you seeing from and what are you seeing?

- Outside/inside/outside
  Allow for open awareness as you let your eyes wander around your space. Let your attention land, and name the thing that you are seeing. Then move your intention inside, notice one feeling or sensation, and name it. And then move outside again, letting your gaze roam, and settling on one object, and then name it to yourself or out loud. Practice this rhythmicity outside, inside, and then back outside a few times a day.

- Horizon awareness (looking up and out, perceiving back body)

  Shift your attention to the level of the horizon and upward. If you work on screens or with your phone, notice when your attention has drawn all the way into your inner world, and lift your gaze and open your peripheral vision.

- Orient in space

  For one minute, look around your space. Slowly look above you, below you, beside you, and behind you. Really take in what you are seeing.

- Eye placement

  Notice where your eyes are in your head. Are they forward toward your face or deep toward the back of your head? Move them forward a bit and notice what happens. And then move them back. Notice what feels more comfortable and what feels foreign. See if you can experiment with allowing your eyes to stay a bit in the direction that feels less normal.

- Eye placement in connection—percentage of attention inside or outside

  Notice where your eyes and attention go when you are relating to different people. When you are talking, do you bring your eyes way forward and lean forward? Do you stay back?

DEVELOP YOUR TIMES VOCABULARY AND FLUENCY (PAGE 53)

- Emotion language

  Elaborate on your emotional vocabulary. Review Appendix 1 (page 213), and experiment with using new words to describe your emotions.

- Sensation language

    Check in at the sensation level with your body for thirty seconds. Notice what sensations arise. Start with opposites—hot or cold? Dense or spacious? Tight or open? Solid or hollow?

    Follow a sensation through the TIMES channels. When you notice the sensation, is it an image that arises? If I didn't know what that sensation was, how would you describe it to me in an image?

- What is your go-to channel? The default channel that your system ends up in on its own?

- What channel feels like your biggest resource, the one that brings you more into wholeness or balance?

- What channel is your growth edge, and do you need practice developing?

STRETCHING INTO PLEASURE (PAGE 79)

- **Blue sensations:** Notice one sensation in your body right now that feels "blue," or pleasurable. Where is it? When you notice, does it expand or diminish?

- **Hold it moments:** The next time someone shares good news with you, can you "hold it" and even accentuate it? Can you celebrate it, and extend the enjoyment and appreciation?

- **Blue sandwich:** This is a variation on inside/outside/inside. Now when you go inside, touch down in blue (land and locate it), and then orient out again.

- **Write down examples of blue to red pendulations** that you notice in your thoughts, sensations, or emotions. Then notice blue to red pendulations in your interactions with others.

MOBILIZING FREEZE RESPONSES (PAGE 103)

- **Breathing/sounding:** Breathe in through your nose, and "hum" or "vu" on your exhales five to fifteen times.

- **Sighing and pandiculating:** Notice your inhales, extend them a little, and then yawn and stretch intentionally on your exhales. Inhale, and then stretch your arms and legs as if you are waking up in the morning. Get into it, and really follow your body's desire to move.

EMBODY THE HUNTER (PAGE 121)

- "Vu" Sequence (Do each step two or three times with ample pauses in between to feel what's happening and track through TIMES)

  * Inhale normally, and on the exhale, make the sound "vu."

  * As you make the sound "vu," open and close your lips like a guppy.

  * As you make the sound "vu," open and close your whole mouth, your whole jaw.

  * As you "vu" and open and close your mouth, open and close your hands as well. The sound "vu" will start to morph.

  * Now turn the jaw movements into growling facial expressions, and turn the opening and closing of the hands into growling.

- Activate Your Inner Jaguar

  * Building on the "vu" sequence, get onto your hands and knees.

* On all fours, rock back and forth, feeling weight on your hands and into your haunches. When you lean forward, feel the backs of your arms light up and engage. Set your sights on imaginary prey.

* Track that prey visually as you stalk, zigzagging toward it. Inhabit the predator. Growl, scratch the ground, feel your energy gathering. Follow your impulses. If words come, say them. If movements come, make them. If emotions arise, let them out.

PRACTICE LIMITS AND BOUNDARIES (PAGE 145)

* **Occupy Your Skin:** Rub your hands against each other, building heat and feeling the surface of the palms of your hands.

* **Yes and No**

  * Where is "yes" located in your body?

  * How do you know when something is a "maybe"?

  * What behaviors/movements, language, or emotions do you notice arising when you say yes, but you really mean no?

* Reprogram default responses in the social nervous system

  * What places or groups of people give you a sense of belonging?

  * Who feels like your tribe?

  * If you notice that your default response is **fitting in**, dare to stand out. Make a list of small ways that you could express yourself more fully. Would that be lipstick? Colorful clothing? Expressing an unpopular opinion? Making a video on social media? Showing a side of yourself that is often hidden? What feels like a manageable risk?

* If you notice that your default response is **fawning**, what would happen if you didn't try to "make everything okay," or manage other people's responses or emotions? What is one situation where you could express disagreement safely?

ACKNOWLEDGING WHERE WE ARE AND DEVELOPING SECURE ATTACHMENT (PAGE 161)

• What **attachment style** do you identify with—anchor, wave, or island?

• From noticing your attachment style, what is one thing you could do to communicate about it, to give someone your code about how you might best receive support or love?

• Pay attention to **greetings and salutations**: hellos and goodbyes. Be deliberate when you enter and exit a room, or enter and exit the house, to greet the other humans.

• What is one relationship you have that feels securely attached, with healthy closeness and consistent contact?

SOMATIC CONVERSATIONS AND EXPANDING CAPACITY (PAGE 181)

• **Somatic Conversation:** Here are some questions to have a somatic conversation with yourself or another.

  * What are you noticing **now**?

  * When you notice that emotion, what are you sensing?

  * *Where* are you sensing that in your body?

  * How would you describe that as an image?

  * When you say _____, I notice _____ in my body.

- Introduce **pauses**, whether in self-pleasure or with a partner. Stay present in the pauses, rather than analyzing.

- **Edging:** While building erotic charge, pause, and then change positions—dance, move, shake, undulate, and distribute that charge all over your body.

- **Communicate the channel** you are in with a partner, and invite them there, or decide to change channels together.

GLOSSARY

Note that the terms are placed in the order in which they appear in the book and are grouped by theme and concept.

Interoception/ Inside Awareness: Your ability to sense, feel, perceive, and name what is happening inside your body.

Exteroception/ Outside Awareness: Your ability to sense and perceive outside your body.

Proprioception: Your ability to sense where your body is, and to locate yourself in space in the here and now.

Capacity: Another way of saying nervous system range, tone, and stamina. How far we can be stretched outside our normal range so that our bandwidth expands and we create a new normal.

Charge: Like a plug into a socket sends charge through a cable, experiences can send a charge through our bodies. Synonym for activation.

Orientation: Knowing where you are in time and space. Can be practiced by allowing yourself to freely look all around the space that you are in.

Activation: External stimulus or input that challenges our capacity, in "good" or "bad" ways.

Window of presence: our level of homeostasis, our M.O., our bandwidth, the range of experiences that we are used to having where we are able to stay present. Could be called our comfort zone, but it's not necessarily comfortable.

Trauma: an experience that is incomplete or undigested in your nervous system. It is not the event itself, whether that was little t or big T, it is how your system was able to move through the experience. It's less about what happened and more about what didn't happen inside your system—what you were or were not able to do, in that moment.

Holding charge: Creating a stronger container and more capacity by sustaining the effects of inputting something outside of our normal range.

Pendulation: The process of oscillating back and forth between two things, for example, swinging from red to blue—from something that feels pleasurable to something that feels painful in your system, from what's working to what's not working, in order to develop capacity and range of experience without getting pulled into a rut or habit.

Titration: Introducing just enough activation, novelty, or challenge so that change can occur, but not so much that the container breaks because of the input. A little at a time. The opposite of catharsis.

Channels: The modes through which we sift and filter our experiences. The five channels are thoughts, images, movements, emotions and sensations or the acronym TIMES.

Coupling: When threads of our experience get tangled or fused together; i.e. every time you smell Polo cologne, you think of your grandfather. Some couplings might be obvious to you, like a song reminding you of a moment in your life. Other couplings are happening beneath our conscious awareness.

Uncoupling: The process of untangling threads that have been knotted together so that we can see each strand for what it is, rather than its associations.

Recoupling: The process of creating the associations and connections that you want to remain. For instance, maybe you have uncoupled secure attachment and care from sex, but you would like to experience secure attachment and sex—so you can go through the process of uncoupling and recoupling.

Upregulation: The process of stimulating the system, moving into a more sympathetic state.

Downregulation: The process of slowing the system, moving into a more parasympathetic state.

Differentiation: Our direct experience of what is ours and what is not ours, discerning what belongs to us and what does not belong to us.

Tracking: Like a hunter finding and following footprints, we learn to distinguish and follow the breadcrumbs of sensations, emotions, thoughts, and images in our body.

Coherence: When our vocal tone, the content of what we are saying, our facial expressions, and body language are all communicating the same thing.

Metabolize: The way that we process, digest, and assimilate an experience. An experience is traumatic when we are not able to metabolize it.

Top-down approach: When we assign meaning through logic and narrative. When we use rational thought to look for solutions.

Bottom-up approach: When we listen to and prioritize what the body is communicating through sensations, emotions, and images, allowing the meaning to unfold.

Blue: Something that registers to us as pleasurable or good.

Red: Something that registers to us as unpleasurable or bad.

Default response: The nervous system stress response—fit in, fawn, fight, flight, freeze—that your nervous system most commonly goes to.

Implicit memory: The memory that lives in our body that may not be obvious or familiar to our rational mind.

Explicit memory: What our cognitive mind remembers and what we are accustomed to labeling as "memory."

Upper limit problem: A problem created by stretching our capacity with good things that then pendulates into conflict or disorganization. If we pay attention to the conflict, we don't notice that the "problem" may be a challenge with handling more intimacy, more money, or more recognition.

"Hold It" Moment: When we experience something good and we hold it in our system—stretching our ability to "hold" the positive as the sensations and feelings expand. A chance to expand our capacity for pleasure.

Edging: Developing sexual capacity by coming close to orgasm and then pausing and distributing the sensation and charge throughout your whole body, playing the edge of orgasm without going over it.

Felt sense: Real time full-body perception and self-location beneath the level of thought. May be communicated through sensations or images.

RECOMMENDED RESOURCES

Somatic Experiencing Trauma Institute: www.traumahealing.org
A global network of somatic practitioners that exists to help people heal trauma through the body. An excellent resource to find a practitioner. Or if you are interested in training, the three-year, eleven-module training is an excellent foundation in somatic work.

Holistic Pelvic Care: www.wildfeminine.com
Tami Lynn Kent is the founder and teacher of Holistic Pelvic Care, a technique designed to restore physical, emotional, and energetic imbalances rooted in the pelvic bowl.

FLO Living: www.floliving.com
Holistic evidence-based support for gynecological and hormonal imbalance, for symptoms like PMS, PCOS, infertility, endometriosis, perimenopause, and missing or irregular periods.

The Fajardo Method of Holistic Biomechanics: www.transformationspdx.com
Nervous system health and biomechanics, which include body structure, alignment, and healthy, supported movement. Individual sessions, group classes, and trainings.

MindLift: www.mindlift.com
Nervous system informed and performance-based breathwork master classes and trainings with Kasper van der Meulen.

Colorado School of Energy Studies: www.energyschool.com
For training in Biodynamic Craniosacral or Polarity Therapy with polyvagal theory in action through touch.

Steamy Chick: www.steamychick.com
Vaginal steaming has long been part of well-woman care all over the world. Steaming can be a positive reparative experience in the healing of birth trauma, losses, gynecological procedures, period pain, or sexual boundary violations.

The Institute of Somatic Sexology: www.instituteofsomaticsexology.com
The premiere training in Sexological Bodywork for bodyworkers, therapists, and yoga teachers who want to become somatic sex educators that also offers a profound learning experience for people interested in their own erotic development.

Rooted: www.rootedandembodied.com
A virtual community and village devoted to co-imagining new ways of belonging and being together as well as dismantling systems of oppression, including white supremacy. Guided study groups and community courses.

Tune In to Children: www.aleduarte.com
With this program and philosophy, Ale Duarte helps parents and educators help children reorganize and rebalance their autonomic nervous systems, starting at the biological and survival level.

Our Breath Collective: www.ourbreathcollective.com
With backgrounds in Wim Hof, Rebirthing, Transformational Breathwork, yogic pranayama, and high-performance breathing, guides lead daily live twelve- to fifteen-minute breath practices to soothe and regulate the nervous system. Also monthly classes and intensives and comprehensive certifications.

The Wheel of Consent: www.bettymartin.org
Simple and radically transformative tools to practice the ways that we communicate and touch each other. The 3-Minute Game is the single most powerful framework I've worked with to practice consent in real time, and therefore radically transform trauma and relational dynamics. When trauma happens through touch, touch is often needed for healing.

FURTHER READING

When my clients ask for resources, these are the books that I point them toward.

ON EMBODIMENT:

Bodyfulness: Somatic Practices for Presence, Empowerment, and Waking Up in This Life by Christine Caldwell (Shambhala, 2018)
Stalking Wild Psoas: Embodying Your Core Intelligence by Liz Koch (North Atlantic, 2019)

ON WOMEN'S SEXUALITY AND CYCLES:

Come as You Are: The Surprising New Science that Will Transform Your Sex Life by Emily Nagoski, PhD (Simon & Schuster, 2015)
In the FLO: Unlock Your Hormonal Advantage and Revolutionize Your Life by Alisa Vitti (HarperOne, 2020)
The Female Brain by Louann Brizendine (Morgan Road Books, 2006)
The Fifth Vital Sign: Master Your Cycles & Optimize Your Fertility by Lisa Hendrickson-Jack (Fertility Friday Publishing, 2019)
Good Sex: Getting Off without Checking Out by Jessica Graham (North Atlantic, 2017)

Wild Feminine: Finding Power, Spirit & Joy in the Female Body by Tami Lynn
Kent (Atira, 2011)
Women's Anatomy of Arousal: Secret Maps to Buried Pleasure by Sheri Wins-
ton (Mango Garden Press, 2009)

ON TRAUMA:

Body Keeps the Score: Brain, Mind, and Body in the Healing for Trauma by
Bessel van der Kolk, PhD (Penguin, 2010)
*The Pocket Guide to the Polyvagal Theory: The Transformative Power of Feel-
ing Safe* by Dr. Stephen Porges (W. W. Norton & Co., 2017)
Waking the Tiger: Healing Trauma by Peter Levine, PhD (North Atlantic
Books, 1997)

ON RACE & SOMATIC ACTIVISM:

Medical Bondage: Race, Gender, and the Origins of American Gynecology by
Deirdre Cooper Owens (University of Georgia Press, 2018)
*My Grandmother's Hands: Racialized Trauma & the Pathway to Mending Our
Hearts and Bodies* by Resmaa Menakem (Central Recovery, 2017)
Pleasure Activism: The Politics of Feeling Good by adrienne maree brown (AK
Press, 2019)

ON ATTACHMENT:

*Attached: The New Science of Adult Attachment and How It Can Help You Find—
and Keep—Love* by Amir Levine and Rachel Heller (TarcherPerigee, 2012)
*Wired for Love: How Understanding Your Partner's Brain and Attachment
Style Can Help You Defuse Conflict and Build a Secure Relationship* by Stan
Tatkin (New Harbinger, 2012)
Strange Situation: A Mother's Journey into the Science of Attachment by Beth-
any Saltman (Ballantine Books, 2020)

ON BIRTH & MOTHERHOOD:

Body Full of Stars: Female Rage and My Passage into Motherhood by Molly
Caro May (Counterpoint, 2019)

The Fourth Trimester: A Postpartum Guide to Healing Your Body, Balancing Your Emotions, and Restoring Your Vitality by Kimberly Ann Johnson (Shambhala, 2017)

Ancient Map for Modern Birth: Preparation, Passage, and Personal Growth for the Childbearing Year by Pam England (Seven Gates Media, 2017)

BIBLIOGRAPHY

Akomolafe, Bayo. *These Wilds Beyond Our Fences: Letters to My Daughter on Humanity's Search for Home*. Berkeley, CA: North Atlantic Books, 2017.

Allione, Tsultrim. *Feeding Your Demons: Ancient Wisdom for Resolving Inner Conflict*. New York, NY: Little, Brown Spark, 2008.

Brizendine, Louann. *The Female Brain*. New York, NY: Morgan Road Books, 2006.

Brody, Karen. *Daring to Rest: Reclaim Your Power with Yoga Nidra Rest Meditation*. Boulder, CO: Sounds True, 2017.

Brogan, Kelly, MD. *A Mind of Your Own: The Truth About Depression and How Women Can Heal Their Bodies to Reclaim Their Lives*. New York, NY: HarperWave, 2016.

brown, adrienne maree. *Emergent Strategy: Shaping Change, Changing Worlds*. Chico, CA: AK Press, 2017.

brown, adrienne maree. *Pleasure Activism: The Politics of Feeling Good*. Chico, CA: AK Press, 2019.

Caldwell, Christine, PhD. *Bodyfulness: Somatic Practices for Presence, Empowerment, and Waking Up in This Life*. Boulder, CO: Shambhala, 2018.

Carney, Scott. *What Doesn't Kill Us: How Freezing Water, Extreme Altitude, and Environmental Conditioning Will Renew Our Lost Evolutionary Strength*. New York, NY: Rodale, 2018.

Chan, Karen B. K. "Blue Fish." February 8, 2015. YouTube video, 2:36. https://www.youtube.com/watch?v=6uyVrWtJDbs.

Chan, Karen B. K. "Jam." January 31, 2013. YouTube video, 5:52. https://www.youtube.com/watch?v=bgd3m-x46JU&t=7s.

Chidi, Erica. *Nurture: A Modern Guide to Pregnancy, Birth, Early Motherhood—and Trusting Yourself and Your Body.* San Francisco: Chronicle Books, 2017.

Chitty, John. *Dancing with Yin and Yang.* Boulder, CO: Polarity Press, 2013.

Dana, Deb. *The Polyvagal Theory in Therapy: Engaging the Rhythm of Regulation.* New York, NY: W. W. Norton, 2018.

Ekman, Paul, PhD. *Emotions Revealed: Recognizing Faces and Feelings to Improve Communication and Emotional Life.* 2nd ed. New York, NY: Holt Paperbacks, 2007.

Ensler, Eve. *In the Body of the World: A Memoir of Cancer and Connection.* New York, NY: Metropolitan Books, 2013.

Feldenkrais, Moshe. *The Potent Self: A Study of Spontaneity and Compulsion.* Berkeley, CA: Frog Books, 2002.

Feldman Barrett, Lisa, PhD. *How Emotions Are Made: The Secret Life of the Brain.* New York, NY: Mariner Books, 2018.

Gonzalez, Nicholas, MD. *Nutrition and the Autonomic Nervous System: The Scientific Foundations of The Gonzalez Protocol.* New York, NY: New Spring Press, 2017.

Graham, Jessica. *Good Sex: Getting Off without Checking Out.* Berkeley, CA: North Atlantic Books, 2017.

Haines, Staci. *The Politics of Trauma: Somatics, Healing, and Social Justice.* Berkeley, CA: North Atlantic Books, 2019.

Heller, Lawrence, PhD, and Aline LaPierre, PsyD. *Healing Developmental Trauma: How Early Trauma Affects Self-Regulation, Self-Image, and the Capacity for Relationship.* Berkeley, CA: North Atlantic Books, 2012.

Hendricks, Gay, PhD. *The Big Leap: Conquer Your Hidden Fear and Take Life to the Next Level.* San Francisco, CA: HarperOne, 2010.

Hendrickson-Jack, Lisa. *The Fifth Vital Sign: Master Your Cycles & Optimize Your Fertility.* Toronto: Fertility Friday Publishing, 2019.

Kantor, Jodi, and Megan Twohey. *She Said: Breaking the Sexual Harassment Story That Helped Ignite a Movement.* New York, NY: Penguin Books, 2019.

Keleman, Stanley. *Your Body Speaks Its Mind.* Berkeley, CA: Center Press, 1981.

Kent, Tami Lynn. *Wild Feminine: Finding Power, Spirit & Joy in the Female Body.* New York, NY: Atria/Beyond Words, 2011.

Koch, Liz. *Stalking Wild Psoas: Embodying Your Core Intelligence.* Berkeley, CA: North Atlantic Books, 2019.

Krans, Kim. *Blossoms and Bones: Drawing a Life Back Together.* San Francisco, CA: HarperOne, 2020.

Levine, Amir, MD, and Rachel S. F. Heller, MA. *Attached: The New Science of Adult Attachment and How It Can Help You Find—and Keep—Love.* New York, NY: TarcherPerigee, 2012.

Levine, Peter A., PhD. *In an Unspoken Voice: How the Body Releases Trauma and Restores Goodness*. Berkeley, CA: North Atlantic Books, 2010.

Levine, Peter A., PhD. *Trauma and Memory: Brain and Body in a Search for the Living Past: A Practical Guide for Understanding and Working with Traumatic Memory*. Berkeley, CA: North Atlantic Books, 2015.

Levine, Peter A, PhD. *Waking the Tiger: Healing Trauma*. Berkeley, CA: North Atlantic Books, 1997.

Lorde, Audre. *Sister Outsider: Essays and Speeches*. Berkeley, CA: Crossing Press, 1984.

May, Molly Caro. *Body Full of Stars: Female Rage and My Passage into Motherhood*. Berkeley, CA: Counterpoint, 2019.

McClain, Dani. *We Live for the We: The Political Power of Black Motherhood*. New York, NY: Bold Type Books, 2019.

Menakem, Resmaa. *My Grandmother's Hands: Racialized Trauma & the Pathway to Mending Our Hearts and Bodies*. Las Vegas, NV: Central Recovery, 2017.

Morin, Jack, PhD. *The Erotic Mind: Unlocking the Inner Sources of Sexual Passion and Fulfillment*. New York, NY: Harper Perennial, 1996.

Nagoski, Emily, PhD. *Come as You Are: The Surprising New Science That Will Transform Your Sex Life*. New York, NY: Simon & Schuster, 2015.

Nestor, James. *Breath: The New Science of a Lost Art*. New York, NY: Riverhead, 2020.

Northrup, Kate. *Do Less: A Revolutionary Approach to Time and Energy Management for Ambitious Women*. Carlsbad, CA: Hay House, 2020.

Owens, Deidre Cooper. *Medical Bondage: Race, Gender, and the Origins of American Gynecology*. Athens, GA: University of Georgia Press, 2018.

Pelmas, Christiane. *Trauma: A Practical Guide to Working with Body and Soul (A Somatic Sex Educator's Handbook)*. Boulder, CO: CreateSpace Independent Publishing Platform, 2017.

Perel, Esther. *Mating in Captivity: Unlocking Erotic Intelligence*. New York, NY: Harper, 2012.

Porges, Stephen W. *The Pocket Guide to the Polyvagal Theory: The Transformative Power of Feeling Safe*. New York, NY: W. W. Norton, 2017.

Rolf, Ida P., PhD. *Rolfing: Reestablishing the Natural Alignment and Structural Integration of the Human Body for Vitality and Well-Being*. Rev. ed. Rochester, VT: Healing Arts Press, 1989.

Rosenberg, Marshall B., PhD. *Nonviolent Communication: A Language of Life*. 2nd ed. Encinitas, CA: Puddledancer Press, 2003.

Rosenberg, Stanley. *Accessing the Healing Power of the Vagus Nerve: Self-Help Exercises for Anxiety, Depression, Trauma, and Autism*. Berkeley, CA: North Atlantic Books, 2017.

Rothschild, Babette. *The Body Remembers: The Psychophysiology of Trauma and Trauma Treatment*. New York, NY: W. W. Norton, 2000.

Saltman, Bethany. *Strange Situation: A Mother's Journey into the Science of Attachment*. New York, NY: Ballantine Books, 2020.

Schnarch, David, PhD. *Secrets of a Passionate Marriage: Keeping Love and Intimacy Alive in Committed Relationships*. New York, NY: W. W. Norton, 2009.

Tatkin, Stan. *Wired for Dating: How Understanding Neurobiology and Attachment Style Can Help You Find Your Ideal Mate*. Oakland, CA: New Harbinger, 2016.

Tatkin, Stan. *Wired for Love: How Understanding Your Partner's Brain and Attachment Style Can Help You Defuse Conflict and Build a Secure Relationship*. Oakland, CA: New Harbinger, 2012.

Thomashauer, Regena. *Pussy: A Reclamation*. Carlsbad, CA: Hay House, 2018.

Van der Kolk, Bessel, MD. *Body Keeps the Score: Brain, Mind, and Body in the Healing for Trauma*. New York, NY: Penguin, 2010.

Vitti, Alisa. *In the FLO: Unlock Your Hormonal Advantage and Revolutionize Your Life*. San Francisco, CA: HarperOne, 2020.

Welch, Claudia, MSOM. *Balance Your Hormones, Balance Your Life: Achieving Optimal Health and Wellness through Ayurveda, Chinese Medicine, and Western Science*. Cambridge, MA: Da Capo, 2011.

Winston, Sheri. *Women's Anatomy of Arousal: Secret Maps to Buried Pleasure*. Kingston, NY: Mango Garden Press, 2009.

INDEX

ABOUT THE AUTHOR

KIMBERLY ANN JOHNSON is a somatic experiencing trauma-resolution practitioner, sexological bodyworker, yoga teacher trainer, birth doula, and single mom. She is out to democratize information that is usually reserved for the highly specialized—how the nervous system and female arousal work, and what healthy sexuality looks like. She is the host of the *Activate Your Inner Jaguar: Sex, Birth and Trauma* podcast with over half a million downloads.

Johnson is the author of the early-mothering classic *The Fourth Trimester: Healing Your Body, Balancing Your Emotions and Restoring Your Vitality* published in seven languages around the world. A sought-after practitioner and lead authority in postpartum health, Johnson has led thousands of women worldwide to heal trauma and feel pleasure through in-person sessions, workshops, and trainings, as well as in her signature online courses, and inspiring global community.

Johnson is known as the "vaginapractor"; her work has been featured in the *New York Times*, *Forbes*, *Vogue*, *New York Magazine*'s The Cut, *Harper's Bazaar*, Today.com, and many more. Her crowning achievement remains her thirteen-year-old Brazilian daughter and partner-in-crime, Cecília.